ROUTLEDGE LIBRARY EDITIONS:
AESTHETICS

Volume 1

AN INTRODUCTION TO AESTHETICS

AN INTRODUCTION TO AESTHETICS

E. F. CARRITT

Routledge
Taylor & Francis Group
LONDON AND NEW YORK

First published in 1949 by Hutchinson's University Library

This edition first published in 2016
by Routledge
2 Park Square, Milton Park, Abingdon, Oxon OX14 4RN

and by Routledge
605 Third Avenue, New York, NY 10017

Routledge is an imprint of the Taylor & Francis Group, an informa business

British Library Cataloguing in Publication Data
A catalogue record for this book is available from the British Library

ISBN: 978-1-138-67507-0 (Set)
ISBN: 978-1-315-56086-1 (Set) (ebk)
ISBN: 978-1-138-65010-7 (Volume 1) (hbk)

Publisher's Note
The publisher has gone to great lengths to ensure the quality of this reprint but points out that some imperfections in the original copies may be apparent.

Disclaimer
The publisher has made every effort to trace copyright holders and would welcome correspondence from those they have been unable to trace.

AN INTRODUCTION TO ÆSTHETICS

by

E. F. CARRITT

HUTCHINSON'S UNIVERSITY LIBRARY
11 Stratford Place, London, W.1
New York Melbourne Sydney Cape Town

THIS VOLUME IS NUMBER 26 IN
HUTCHINSON'S UNIVERSITY LIBRARY

Printed in Great Britain by
William Brendon and Son, Ltd.
The Mayflower Press (late of Plymouth)
at Bushey Mill Lane
Watford, Herts.

CONTENTS

PREFATORY NOTE

I trust that readers will not be deterred by the forbidding title of "Appendices." I believe they are in some ways the most useful part of this book. They provide in concise form the data on which the conclusions reached in the more consecutive text are based, and by which they must be tested. The only data for an æsthetic theory are æsthetic experiences, either first-hand or at second-hand from presumably sensitive minds.

My pupil, Mr. J. Hartland-Swann, and my brother-in-law, Mr. J. L. Etty, have both read my typescript and given me valuable criticism and suggestions.

ANALYSIS

I. The Subject of Æsthetics

§1. Subject matter of æsthetics.

§2. The problem of æsthetics. It cannot establish a criterion or rules for production and appreciation.

§3. Æsthetics cannot directly alter our æsthetic experiences but only helps us to understand them.

§4. Æsthetics cannot tell us what we *mean* by "beautiful" or "æsthetic."

§5. It might tell us what other common quality (if any) all æsthetic experiences or beautiful things have, which, though we were not thinking of it, made them such.

§6. If we ask this question about beautiful things the best answer seems to be that they are the sensible things which please us by their significance or meaning.
(Not all significant or meaningful things are beautiful. Only sensible things or sensuous images, and only those whose meaning is natural or immediate not conventional.)

§7. But if this answer be accepted the question ought to have been asked about æsthetic experiences rather than beautiful things since things have no meaning in themselves. We mean something by them or read a meaning into them.

§8. Beauty, then, though we generally *mean* to attribute it to objects, is wrongly so attributed, as are "strangeness," "pleasantness," etc.

§9. Other arguments for the subjective character of beauty besides its significance:
- (*a*) Beauty largely depends upon secondary qualities which depend on our organs.
- (*b*) Even the primary qualities of shape and size look very different under a microscope.
- (*c*) The actual conformation of physical things is probably very different from anything we can possibly see.

§10. It might be said beauty is a real quality of our sensa,

though those indeed are conditioned by our organs, memories, health, interest, etc.
But of two mental images, qualitatively indistinguishable, one might be more or less significant to me, or to other persons, or differently so, at different times.

§11. It will be begging no question as to the objective reality of beauty if we look for grounds of æsthetic experience rather than of beauty.

II.—Good and Bad Taste

§1. Is it possible to speak of good and bad taste if no objects are really beautiful?

§2. Of two men one may have an æsthetic experience and the other none in face of the same object, or they may have æsthetic experiences with different degrees of intensity and purity.

§3. It is difficult to estimate the purity of one's own taste, impossible that of another; but we can guess.

§4. Some objects are more apt to stimulate æsthetic experience in persons of a given nature or culture, but genius overcomes obstacles. The perfect æsthete would not be human.

III.—What is Signified by Beauty?

§1. Not all significant objects or symbols are æsthetic. They may signify historical, scientific or moral facts.

§2. It has been held that æsthetic experience is "sensuous knowledge," which is sometimes regarded as inferior, sometimes as superior to reason.

§3. "Sensuous knowledge" here seems identical with wishful thinking. Art can be either edifying or debauching to inartistic minds.

§4. It is not true that fine æsthetic taste or even creative genius either supersedes moral thinking or ensures moral practice or is morally better than conscientious conduct.

§5. Yet we condemn some art as "insincere," "untrue," "affected." Genuine æsthetic experience might be the finding or making some sensuous object or image *expressive* of one's own feelings or moods. (If it were *descriptive* it would be psychology.) Art is the communication of such expression by the fashioning of some sensible material.

§6. Application of "emotional expressiveness" to various arts.

§7. And to natural beauties.

§8. The expression—theory makes beauty subjective, but can allow differences of pure and impure, faint and profound æsthetic experiences.

§9. Differences inborn or acquired must determine men's different interpretations,

§10. But may allow of equally good æsthetic experiences. Analogies with the affectionate and moral experiences.

IV.—Formal and Representative Art

§1. Former intolerance of any art without an important or interesting subject matter.

§2. Present intolerance of art with such or any subject matter, i.e. in any degree representative. This seems an even less plausible sectarianism.

§3. Pure unrepresentative form is highly æsthetic (i.e. expressive) to us all in architecture and music. We cannot say it may not be so to some people in miniatures or in speech. Analogy from moral experience.

§4. To deny that either can be æsthetically expressive to those of different temperament or culture is dogmatic.

§5. Kant on free and dependent beauty.

§6. Inconsistent modern tendencies.

V.—Kinds of Beauty

§1. Has all æsthetic experience a common and peculiar nature? If so, are there distinguishable species each with its specific difference? or is it an *infima species*?

§2. Various specifications have been suggested on various principles of division.

§3. Their inconsistency suggests that the attempt was mistaken. Further sub-divisions possible but unconvincing. The most plausible distinction is between naturalistic and formal art.

§4. Either of these might be the more expressive to persons of a given temperament or culture.

§5. Words used to denote species of beauty really indicate elements necessary in some degree to every æsthetic experience, elements one of which may unduly predominate and so lead to a deviation from perfection.
§6. If beauty is the achievement of expression of emotion, either the expressiveness or the expressed may be somewhat wanting.
§7. Less ambitious classifications are more useful.
§8. Degrees of complexity in the arts.
§9. The film.
§10. The vice of classification.

VI.—Expression

§1. Expression distinguished from sign and symptom.
§2. Language as eminently expressive.
§3. Expression as distinguished from symbol.
§4. Expression as distinguished from stimulation.
§5. Expression as distinguished from communication.
§6. Propaganda and argument.
§7. The artist's deliberate intention is irrelevant. We can only judge our experience of his work.
§8. Communication and expression.
§9. Creation and technique.

VII.—Emotion

§1. The second term of the definition also needs elucidation. It has been criticized (A) as too wide, (B) as too narrow.
§2. (A) This has been held on two grounds. (i) On the ethical ground that some emotions are too bad to be expressed. But if they *are* human emotions most of us can imagine them in an æsthetic experience. Disinterested love of evil is not human.
§3. (ii) On the psychological ground that localized sensations, and perhaps some others, cannot in fact be æsthetically expressed. This seems true, but these are not emotions, they cannot be imagined in tranquillity.
§4. (B) It is held, conversely, that other experiences than those of emotion are æsthetic. It seems true that no sane human experience is purely intellectual or emotional

or conative. But we can distinguish the predominant element. We can read a poem for its doctrine or for the expression of the emotion generated by that doctrine. Only the latter experience is æsthetic.

VIII.—Didactic and Protreptic Art

§1. Is an æsthetic experience ever predominantly expressive of (A) thought or (B) will? (Mere sensation has been excluded.)

§2. (A) The truth-value of poetry is often confused with its beauty value. Many of the emotions expressed depend upon beliefs held. Such beliefs may be contradictory but the expressions equally beautiful; and the expression of belief, true or false, however perfect, is often not beautiful.

§3. (B) The moderns confuse art less often with philosophy or theology than with sincere propaganda. This implies that the encouragement in others, whether by argument or appeals to passion, of a policy really acted on by the artist is æsthetic expression. This implies censorship and neglects imagination. The objections to it are:

(i) We can appreciate the expression of conflicting enthusiasms.
(ii) Much propaganda is not beautiful.
(iii) The artist need not actually adopt a policy when he imagines the enthusiasm of its adherents. Nor need his hearers.

§4. Propaganda in the graphic arts.

§5. Escapism.

IX.—The Tasks of Criticism

§1. Historical criticism.

§2. Discovery, restoration and interpretation.

§3. Æsthetic criticism proper aims at extending and purifying æsthetic experience.

§4. Methods of criticism.

§5. Artists as critics.

X.—The Genesis of Æsthetic Expressions

§1. Complexity of the problem.

§2. (i) *Physical* stimulus.

XVI.—[illegible] Speech in Poetry

APPENDIX

[illegible]

[illegible] Successive Poems

CHAPTER I

THE SUBJECT OF ÆSTHETICS

§1. The subject of æsthetic philosophy or reflection or analysis is obviously æsthetic experience. Its presupposition, therefore, is that rational sensitive beings such as men have a set of experiences pretty clearly distinguishable from others. They are those which we usually express by some such phrase as "How beautiful!" (or "How ugly!") and not by "How true!", "How good!", "How useful!", nor even "How pleasant!" (nor "How false, evil, useless or painful"). No doubt æsthetic experiences are as a rule predominantly pleasant, but in those that are described as tragic there is an essentially painful element, and there are many pleasant experiences, such as a warm bath or a healthy digestive process, which we should not call beautiful unless with conscious humour or exaggeration. We seldom use language carefully and should sometimes loosely speak of a beautiful steak or experiment or operation, but on reflection should admit that such usage was loose.

Dr. Johnson[1] defined beauty as "that assemblage of graces or proportions of parts which pleases the eye." He should have added "or ear or imagination" unless he was excluding poetry and music. What sorts of objects or qualities, then, are apt to excite in us those experiences which we should most deliberately express by the word beautiful or some cognate term (pretty, charming, lovely, sublime or ugly, hideous, and the like)? The *qualities* we should with confidence name would unquestionably be colours, shapes, sounds, and combinations or patterns of these; and we might perhaps add some smells and tastes and even some sensations of touch. It is hard to exclude any class of *objects* from the sphere of possible æsthetic experience; but those which seem specially apt to excite it are human bodies and faces, animals, vegetables,

[1]*Dictionary*, eleventh edition, 1799.

B

sky, water, fire, and the lie of the land.[1] These are all natural objects, but they may be more or less exactly reproduced or suggested by human agency, which may also produce the qualities or patterns mentioned above, as in arabesque, architecture, dancing and musical performance. Human agency, moreover, may produce physical symbols, such as spoken or written words or musical scores, which though not themselves describable as beautiful are apt to stimulate, in those who know the symbolism, mental imagery which is.

I think this group of experiences is as properly classed together and distinguished from others as the classes which we call moral, intellectual, conative or appetitive experiences. It may be impossible, or at least not known to occur, that a creature should have the æsthetic experience who was incapable of the others or should have the moral or intellectual while incapable of the æsthetic, and yet all are *distinguishable.* We can surely conceive of the appetitive experience as occurring alone. Some of the others may not be *separable.*

There certainly are some border-line experiences which we should be uncertain whether to class simply as æsthetic and as differing from obvious instances only in *degree* of beauty, or as different from the æsthetic experience in kind, though superficially similar, or again as distinguishable *kinds* of the æsthetic. Perhaps the most strikingly dubious of these are the experiences of the ludicrous, which we express by laughter or by phrases like "How funny!" (or "What a bad joke!") and those of the "sublime," when we are apt to say, "How grand!" (or "How high falutin!" or "How ridiculous!"). But such nice discriminations, which will have to be discussed, need not invalidate our main contention that there is a real class of æsthetic experiences.[2]

§2. If then the subject of æsthetic philosophy is our æsthetic experiences, what do we think it will teach us about them? What is "the problem of æsthetics"?

I think most people approach the subject from controversial criticism of particular works or schools of art. They

[1]Among artifacts produced solely with a view to utility perhaps the most generally apt to seem beautiful have been sailing vessels.

[2]*See* Chapter VII.

hope and expect that they will be able to discover an indubitable definition or criterion of beauty from which judgments on the work of particular schools or artists can be demonstratively deduced. The same would then be true about natural beauties, though this is not so generally remarked; it would be possible to prove that the seventeenth century was right or wrong in thinking mountains merely "horrid," and even to settle definitely the more definite question, eagerly debated in the eighteenth century, whether Dovedale or Borrowdale were the more beautiful.[1]

Such hopes, I believe, are destined to disappointment; and surely they were founded on a mistake. The only datum from which æsthetic philosophy can start is the æsthetic experience of mankind, primarily the philosopher's own and indirectly that of other people so far as he can confidently trust their reports. That is the method I propose to follow. To deny that an experience is æsthetic out of deference to an æsthetic theory, though careful introspection testifies to its æsthetic nature, would be to tamper with the data on which alone the theory could be founded. It would be like denying the existence of a visible planet because your astronomical system did not allow of it. This illusion is perhaps now mainly confined to beginners in æsthetics, but it was characteristic of most æsthetic philosophy in the eighteenth century, a century which painted pictures by the book and devoutly believed in "the rules of old discovered not devised" by Aristotle, Horace, "Longinus," Vitruvius, Palladio and their followers down to Boileau and Lessing, and which condemned works of art or nature that did not conform to these. The most notorious of such rules, because the most definite, were the unities of time and place, according to which you could discover by the clock whether a tragedy were good or bad, or at least whether it had a fatal flaw. Other rules of art were so vague as to be manageable: "the work of art must have a certain size; it must have a beginning, a middle, and an end; it must have a unity of subject"; or "it must have symmetry and proportion and harmony." But there will be as much dispute whether it has symmetry, harmony and proportion, which are all æsthetic,

[1]*London Magazine*, October, 1778.

not scientific terms, as whether it has beauty. Most of these rules were reached *a priori*. In modern times similar precepts have been more reasonably based empirically. Hogarth maintained that the serpentine or spiral line was the line of grace, and the pyramid the most beautiful mass; Fechner, on somewhat better evidence, that most men gave the preference among rectangular figures to "the golden section" whose sides were in the proportion 21 : 34. But it had at once to be admitted that, in ordinary æsthetic experiences, association and context, which in the psychological experiments are as far as possible excluded, play a far greater part than geometrical or arithmetical relations.

§3. Æsthetics then can do little or nothing to improve our taste. Even if it could prove to me, as it cannot, that a play which keeps the unity of time is more beautiful than Macbeth, I might still prefer Macbeth, and could merely be driven to the insincere confession that my taste was bad; all that could really be proved would be that it was different from the taste of many or most people or people of some particular set.

What then can æsthetics do for us? It cannot increase our æsthetic enjoyments, and should not I think be allowed to direct them to different objects, but it can help us to understand them. Its object, like that of all philosophy (φιλοσοφία), is to satisfy curiosity, and if we have no curiosity about such subjects it will give us little satisfaction. For some people the satisfaction of their curiosity about æsthetic experience is almost as valuable as that experience itself, and confusion of mind almost as grievous as ugliness. Hardly anyone who has taken part in amateur discussions on artistic topics can have escaped irritation alike at his own muddleheadedness and at that of the rest. Similar discussions, by practised thinkers, if not conclusive, are more profitable; words are used in the same senses and there is less misunderstanding and irrelevancy if not much more agreement.

§4. There seem to be two main questions which æsthetics might be expected to answer. The first is "What do we *mean* when we call things beautiful?" which is to ask for a definition that gives the meaning of a name.[1] But this question cannot

[1]Aristotle, *Post. Analyt.* 93b.

be answered. If we were to say, "We mean that they give us a certain kind of pleasure" it is still required to know *what* kind, and if the answer be "æsthetic pleasure" we are only repeating the undefined term beautiful in another language.[1] All other attempts to explain the meaning of the word fail: for instance, "Beautiful means that whose contemplation is good" or "whose contemplation makes us better men" or "whose contemplation has survival value" or "whose contemplation gives us an immediate knowledge which might also be reached by scientific argument." Any one of these statements might conceivably be true if it began with the words "Beautiful *is* that which . . ." but when it begins "Beautiful *means* that which . . ." we see at once that it is not true. We at once ask ourselves "Is it not at least intelligible to ask whether beautiful things *are* all of that nature?" and since we must answer "yes," it clearly was not what we *meant*. We can illustrate this by an analogous example. If we ask "What is meant by blue?" and are answered "Blue means such and such a brain movement set up by the stimulation of our optic nerves by such and such light vibrations," we should at once know by introspection that this was not what we had *meant* when we called a violet blue.[2] Nothing of the sort was in our minds. If on the other hand we had been told that blue means a certain kind of visual sensation we should still want to know what kind and what was meant by visual. There are many terms whose meaning cannot be defined without tautology except by what is rather absurdly called ostensive definition; I might point to some violets, flags, ribbons and sky patches and say, "That is what I meant by blue"; to Miss Gunning, a mountain, a poem, an arabesque, and say "That is what I mean by beautiful." But this would not be definition. I cannot define the meaning of beauty, goodness, duty, pleasure, necessitation, causality, relationship, quality, though I could define what I mean and what I think most people to-day and in this country mean by, say, a "steam-engine."

§5. There is, however, a different question which æsthetics

[1]Not Greek but Baumgartenian German.

[2]This may be called the "heterogeneous fallacy." It is called by Aristotle a μεταβασις εἰς ἀ'λλο λένος

might more plausibly be expected to answer: Is there any other common quality which all our æsthetic experiences (or all beautiful things) have, in virtue of which, though we may not have thought of it, they are æsthetic (or beautiful)? I have put the former and more clumsy expression first, because the second and more natural one, which I have put in brackets, unconsciously begs an important question with which it will be better to begin.

If we ask the question in the second or bracketed way, our natural answer will probably be that beautiful things are those which it is pleasant to see or hear, but that the pleasure they give us has a peculiar quality different both from the satisfaction of an appetite and also from merely passive titillation; a quality which has been described as significance or meaning. This is perhaps clearest in the literary arts, but is also apparent in most painting and sculpture, and hardly less so in music, architecture and dancing. All of these are the works of artists who meant to convey something to us in them, something which can, not improperly, be called a meaning. What the artists meant they may be unable to express in any other way; if they could have put it into vulgar prose they would not have troubled to write verses or this particular and carefully selected prose, nor to paint, carve and compose. So, too, we can sometimes convey by a smile or a handshake something not fully expressible in words. Actors know this well.

When we turn to natural beauties it is not so easy to see how they can be said to have meaning or significance; yet the conviction that they have is so strong that theologians have been tempted to hazard the conjecture that "nature is the art of God." But there is clearly a sense in which objects that were never given a meaning, such as a dead child's toys, may have one for us, if not æsthetic, at least by association. How stormy sunsets, the starlit sky and the riding moon, forests, waterfalls and the sea came to have for men their almost universal significance is a fascinating question which we shall discuss. All of them exact close attention from primitive man for practical reasons; all by their change and motion seem analogous with man's life and mind. The most difficult case is with the rather stolid beauties of sheer line and mass, but modern theories have maintained that we read into them our own physical experiences; we certainly speak of a springing arch, dancing lines and a restful pattern; but all this will need more detailed treatment.[1]

§6. If we think that the most striking common characteristic of all things called beautiful is their significance, we must remind ourselves that this is not peculiar to them. $\sqrt{4}$ and 4x are significant symbols but not beautiful nor suggestive of beautiful imagery, and so are some words and sentences and gestures and mechanical signals such as a siren. We should therefore have to add that to be called beautiful, a thing must be significant in virtue of its sensible character or of the sensuous images it arouses in our minds, which is to say that the symbolism must be natural or "second nature," not conventional or accidental. A poem is significant by its sounds and the images it immediately evokes; if translated into other words it would either have a different beauty or none.[2] $\sqrt{4}$ can be just as well expressed as "the square root of four" or in French. We may have to go further yet to find a completely exhaustive and exclusive differentiation of beauty, but the twofold character of sensuous significance is enough for our present purpose.

§7. If we are right in thinking that beauty is always significant, then we must have been mistaken in thinking that it is, in the strict sense, a quality of the objects to which we attributed it. The meaning of the word "*lit*" whether as written or pronounced is different for the French and the English, and neither can be said to be the true or actual meaning which it really has. The word "ball" in the sentence "I will give you a ball" may have different meanings in different contexts; a speaker might "mean" it in one sense and the hearer understand it in the other; in fact, as has been well said: "Things do not mean, it is we who mean by them." "The word is halfe his that speaketh, and halfe his that hearkeneth unto it," says Montaigne in Florio's translation. The same is true of symbols other than verbal, such as red flags, blue ribbons and algebraical

[1]*See* Chapter X.
[2]But *see* Chapter XV.

signs; their meaning is a relation between the symbol and the persons who use or understand it on any occasion. The meaning of the symbol O is not a quality of it, as its oval shape is, but a relation it often has to the minds of mathematicians and cricketers.

§8. If then beauty is or depends upon significance, and the meaning or significance of anything for you or me depends upon our nature or on acquired associations with the thing, "its beauty" is not a quality it really has but only a capacity for becoming significant in a certain way to me or to you. We use many words in ways which grammatically would seem to ascribe qualities to objects or events, though we do not really intend to do so. When we call a thunderstorm "unexpected" we merely mean that we had not expected it, and we are not at all disturbed to discover that it was confidently predicted by the meteorologists last night. The optical illusions of eighteenth-century landscape-gardening are "surprising" the first time we experience them, but subsequently merely "tiresome," though they have not changed. By other words we do sometimes unreflectively intend to ascribe a quality, and only on consideration decide that we were wrong. Such words are, for instance, "pleasant," "sweet," "harmonious," "loud," "dazzling," "sad-coloured," "blue."

§9. This reminds us of the second differentiating character we suggested for experiences of beauty. Not only had they to be significant but sensuously significant. A great part of our experiences of beauty depends upon arrangements of colours and sounds, usually described as "secondary qualities," but more properly not as qualities of physical things at all, but sensations or "sensa" dependent upon the presence and condition of bodily organs in ourselves. No doubt there is some real quality or movement in objects which, given the presence of light and of suitable optic nerves, will excite in a consciousness the sensation of redness, but this real quality is not what we call beautiful and is not one that we have ever seen even under a microscope. Moreover, some things beautiful to our normal eyesight quite cease to be so when sufficiently magnified, or assume a very different beauty. Even the actual shape of a cube and the texture of its surface, not to mention the electrons of which it is really composed, are very different from what, as we say, "we see."

§10. We should be driven then to say that it is not physical things which are properly to be called beautiful but only our "ideas" of them, the "sensa" which we have in perceiving or remembering them or which we construct by combination of remembered sensa; and what these sensa are will depend not only upon the acuteness of our senses or the retentiveness of our memory but upon the degree and direction of our interest, which is determined in many ways. A proof-reader may "see" different ink patterns on a page of a novel from those "seen" by one absorbed in the story.

It might seem then that though we cannot properly ascribe beauty to physical things we can ascribe it to our images of them whether perceptual or imaginary. But if we recall what was said about the significance of beauty this will require modification. Of two mental images, whether perceptual or reproductive, which I have at different times and which are qualitatively indistinguishable, one may be very much more "significant" to me than the other. I may look twice at the same picture or landscape from the same angle and in a similar light and even with the same attentiveness, yet have very different æsthetic experiences, or on one occasion none at all. These differences may depend on something I have heard, seen or been through in the interval or upon my momentary mood and preoccupations or even on the fact that I have just had a swim and my tea. We can only say of the image what we said of the object: that it (or, more accurately, any image exactly like it) is capable of stimulating in me or anybody like me a certain æsthetic experience. I have had many dream or fancy pictures as well as perceptions which I could not call beautiful or ugly; they had for me no æsthetic significance.

§11. It will be wiser then to begin by considering the nature of æsthetic experience rather than to beg an important question by talking about beautiful objects or even beautiful images. "It seems impossible to conceive objects themselves to be endowed with more than a particular order of parts, and with powers, or an affinity to our perceptive faculties, thence arising; . . . surely order and regularity are more properly the causes of beauty than beauty itself."[1]

[1]R. Price, *Review of the Principal Questions in Morals* (1757). Cf. Kant, *Critique of Judgment* (trnsl. Bernard) §9. "Beauty apart from relation to our feeling is itself nothing," Rashdall, *Theory of Good and Evil*, I.vi note, and Ross, *The Right and the Good*, pp. 118–31.

CHAPTER II

GOOD AND BAD TASTE

§1. A serious objection may be made to the argument of the preceding chapter on the ground that we seem to have made beauty "subjective," that is to say, wholly dependent on the idiosyncrasy of the person who experiences it, and that, as one man's meat is another's poison, we could not dispute about taste. Yet we are incorrigibly convinced that there is such a thing as bad, vulgar taste, and most of us try to improve our own. Is it possible to defend such judgments consistently with the view that beauty is not a quality of things but is the projection into them of our own æsthetic experience, which is conditioned by our physical organization and by our past history and the associations that give the object significance? Take a very simple case: One man distempers his room dead white and another cream colour; I think we should hesitate to say that either taste was better. But if one of them confessed that the only reasons he could see for a choice of colour were durability, cheapness and hygiene, we should say he was, in this matter, absolutely without taste. If the only decoration he could think of were pornographic or sadistic we should pass the same sentence on him æsthetically and might add that morally he was reprehensible. If all that occurred to him were to adorn his room with busts and photographs of Lenin, Hitler or Churchill we might either admire or deplore his politics but should say he had no taste. If he scrawled texts or equations or charitable appeals on the distemper we might applaud him as a Christian, a mathematician or a philanthropist but condemn him as an artist.

§2. These are extreme instances in which practical, moral or scientific interests seem to have completely displaced the æsthetic; but even in extreme instances it is seldom possible to be sure of another's experience. It is conceivable that the one man was not stimulating his sexual desires, but genuinely delighting in the contemplation of what seemed to him lovely shapes and colours expressive of natural vitality and passion; that the second was no propagandist or victim of propaganda, but saw in his busts the expression of courage, enthusiasm, patriotism, or of ambition, satanic pride, and indomitable will; that the third was æsthetically moved by the poetry, if not the calligraphy, of the texts. The equations and the appeals are perhaps hardest to palliate; might the former express not so much mathematical truth as the triumph of discovery, and the appeals not so much the desire to get our money as the joy in well-doing? It seems unlikely.

§3. Less simple cases are naturally even harder to judge. Novelty is stimulating, for we are all apt to be bored; familiarity is restful for we are all apt to be lazy; and these two weaknesses infect all our activities, intellectual, moral, and æsthetic. But perhaps no counterfeit æsthetic experience is so obvious as that of the man who only likes what is old or what is the latest novelty or the latest archaism. No taste is more worthless than one confined to plays that are all the rage, or to the book of the year, or to the picture exhibition which is a *succès de scandale*, the chatter of all the studios and bitterly controverted in the Press. To be merely and eagerly in the fashion shows little taste in dress. Yet here again it is impossible to be quite certain about other people and difficult about oneself. It admittedly requires as much talent to appreciate the poetry or painting of an age whose history and civilization are unknown to us as to accept the innovations of original genius. There may be adults so childishly engrossed in the passing moment that they can only enter into the topical representations of their own set; we cannot tell if they are really moved by them or only snobbish. When Marianne in *Sense and Sensibility* says "Nay, mamma, if he is not to be animated by Cowper!" I feel sure she had some vivid æsthetic experiences but suspect their range was narrow. Edward himself may have had less keen ones but they were more catholic. Elinor diagnoses him acutely: " 'I suspect that to avoid one kind of affectation Edward here falls into another. Because he believes many people pretend to more admiration for the beauties of nature than they really feel, and is disgusted with such pretensions, he affects greater indifference and less discrimination in viewing them himself than he possesses. He is fastidious and will have an affectation of his own.' 'It is very true,' said Marianne, 'that admiration of landscape scenery has become a mere jargon. Everybody pretends to feel and tries to describe with the taste and elegance of him[1] who first defined what picturesque beauty was' . . . 'I am convinced,' said Edward, 'that you really feel all the delight in a fine prospect which you profess to feel. But in return your sister must allow me to feel no more than I profess. I like a fine prospect but not on picturesque principles . . . a troop of tidy happy villagers please me better than the finest banditti in the world.' Marianne looked with amazement at Edward, with compassion at her sister. Elinor only laughed." I do not remember any neater dialectic of taste than is scattered in Jane Austen; perhaps because I have some sympathy with Edward and much with Elinor. Change the terms of art and the story is true of our own or any day.

§4. There may then be more or less pure and vivid æsthetic experiences in face of various perceptions or imaginations, and the purity and vividness do not entirely depend on what is perceived or imagined, though some objects may be more apt to stimulate than others. If this is so, it might seem that the ideal æsthetic genius would have pure and vivid æsthetic experiences of the favourable kind in all his perceptions and recollections or imaginary combinations of nature. He would find all natural objects beautiful; he would only find ugly what he took to be human products evincing impure taste or complete indifference in their authors. And I am apt to think that the more genuinely æsthetic experiences a man had, in face of no matter what stimulus, the more æsthetic he would be and the better his taste. But a pure æsthete would be inhuman, since his æsthetic experiences could only be invariably pure if he had no passions to disturb them, no affections or enmities, no greed or desire, no politics or religion or love

[1]Probably Uvedale Price, *Essays on the Picturesque*, 1794, "roughness and sudden variation joined to irregularity," or W. Gilpin, *Picturesque Beauty*, 1792. Cf. Payne Knight, *Principles of Taste*, 1805, and Peacock, *Headlong Hall*, 1816; also Hussey, *The Picturesque* for a history of the craze. *See* Maria Edgeworth, *The Absentee* for examples.

of truth. We may find reason to think that for such a being none of his experiences could really be æsthetic at all, since it is hard to see what they could æsthetically signify or express. For the very emotions which when felt disturb æsthetic experiences are those which in tranquillity it contemplates. He would only write a sonnet on the sonnet; he would only criticize the more or less impure art of others, like the man who "knows all about art but does not know what he likes."

There is, then, a class of experiences genuinely æsthetic, though not all experiences for which this character is claimed possess it or not in its purity; and those which do so may differ in vivacity. And we are mistaken when we attribute to the objects which stimulate even the best of such experiences in ourselves a quality called beauty, or when we say that those who are stimulated to such experiences by other objects and not by ours are wrong. But as all men have human nature in common, there is much agreement among all men, and more among those who share a common civilization.

CHAPTER III

WHAT IS SIGNIFIED BY BEAUTY?[1]

§1. Æsthetic experiences seem all to be sense-perceptions or sensuous images with a certain significance, but many experiences which fulfil these two conditions are not æsthetic. Can we say what the nature of the significance must be if they are to deserve the name? Sense-perceptions and memory images are significant of some perceived reality, though they may of course be more or less illusory; but sensa may have no æsthetic quality either favourable or unfavourable, and memory images follow suit. It is generally admitted that the significance of æsthetic experiences is not scientific or historical in the usual sense of those words. A bare narrative, a mathematical equation, a map or a model may give me scientific information if it is correct, but to ask of any æsthetic experience whether it is true of the physical world, now or in the past or future, is irrelevant. A sentence may give me moral or philosophical information, as that we have an obligation not to break our promises or that there are some facts of which knowledge is impossible for the human mind, and it has been held at different times and is still sometimes maintained that æsthetic experiences give us truth about moral or metaphysical facts "in a sensuous form." This needs elucidation.

§2. The contention has taken two forms. One is that the æsthetic experience gives us a vague or incommunicable kind of awareness which requires to be clarified and certified by discursive thinking, much as a child might be said to "feel" that a certain woman was its mother and its sure protector, and would come to a "knowledge" of these facts by experience and by reflection. On this view, which was sometimes adumbrated by Plato[2] and by Hegel among others, the æsthetic

[1]For a fuller treatment of some of the distinctions in this and the next chapter *see* Hospers, *Meaning and Truth in the Arts.*

[2]*Symposium*, 210–11.

experience is a kind of propædeutic or stepping-stone to philosophy, and would be no longer valued when the higher stage had been reached. The other view, more common among artists and mystics, is that the æsthetic experience is a vehicle of truth superior to rational thought, or the only one attainable on the most important matters.

> I felt the sentiment of Being spread
> O'er all that moves and all that seemeth still;
> O'er all that, lost beyond the reach of thought
> And human knowledge, to the human eye
> Invisible, yet liveth to the heart;
> . . . Wonder not
> If high the transport, great the joy I felt
> Communing in this sort through earth and heaven
> With every form of creature, as it looked
> Towards the Uncreated with a countenance
> Of adoration, with an eye of love.
> . . . O Nature! Thou hast fed
> My lofty speculations; and in thee,
> For this uneasy heart of ours, I find
> A never failing principle of joy
> And purest passion.[1]

and again:

> One impulse from a vernal wood
> May teach you more of man;
> Of moral evil and of good,
> Than all the sages can.[2]

This has been expressed by the phrase that beauty is the vehicle of "transcendental feeling"[3] and it has been dramatically put by Browning: "The rest may reason and welcome: 'tis we musicians know."[4] But so far as poems are taken at their face value to make statements about reality, or so far as the

[1]Wordsworth, *The Prelude*, II 401–50.
[2]Ibid., *The Tables Turned.*
[3]Stewart, *The Myths of Plato, see* Appendix A. "A solemn sense of Timeless Being."
[4]*Abt Vogler.*

æsthetic experiences stimulated by music and painting or by autumn, sunset and roses are supposed to give us information about reality, it is indubitable that such statements and informations may contradict one another.

> Vanity of vanities, all is vanity.[1]

is as poetical as

> Underneath are the everlasting arms.[2]

> From too much love of living,
> From hope and fear set free,
> We thank with brief thanksgiving
> Whatever gods may be
> That no life lives for ever;
> That dead men rise up never;
> That even the weariest river
> Winds somewhere safe to sea.[3]

This is fine poetry, and so is the *Ode on Intimations of Immortality*:[4]

> Hence in a season of calm weather
> Though inland far we be,
> Our souls have sight of that immortal sea
> Which brought us hither.[4]

If the last quotation but one conveys "truth" in any usual sense of the word, the last would only convey delusive

> thoughts whose very sweetness yieldeth proof
> That they were born for immortality.[5]

§3. In fact, it is difficult to distinguish "transcendental feeling" from "wishful thinking" which notoriously may be untrue, though it may also be true. The kinds of conviction

[1]*Ecclesiastes*, i.2.
[2]*Deuteronomy*, xxxiii. 27.
[3]Swinburne, *The Garden of Proserpine.*
[4]Wordsworth.
[5]Ibid., *Inside of King's Chapel.*

born in us by certain drugs or stimulants, or political enthusiasm or mob-oratory or beauty, though differing from one another, are all different from knowledge of external facts. That we are subject to these moods is certainly a very interesting fact which may have important implications about our own nature and therefore indirectly about the nature of the universe, but the knowledge so implied would have no æsthetic character; it would be psychology or science or metaphysics.

When the view put forward is that in æsthetic experience we attain *moral* truth the arguments are naturally similar, since the truth about goodness and obligations is truth; there are again two forms of the doctrine. The first is to be found in Plato[1] who thinks that familiarity with the beauties of nature and of formal art somehow predisposes the mind to morality. Of course he also advocates for this purpose the use of carefully moralized fables and poems, and this is the line commonly taken in the sixteenth and seventeenth centuries,[2] and reappearing in Tolstoy.[3] But this is beside the point; it would not be beauty as such, nor even imitative art as such, that would give us moral truth, nor necessarily even the most beautiful imitative art[4] that would be most effective. All that is true in this theory is that artistic beauty can be used for moralizing as well as for debauching men's conduct; it is pleasant and can be used to make anything attractive. For the more serious and genuinely æsthetic doctrine that beauty in nature or formal art predisposes the mind to morality I do not know what can be said. I should not expect the inhabitants of Athens or Venice or Oxford or Switzerland to be more honest, brave, industrious or temperate than those of Pittsburg or the Potteries. On the other side it has been pointed out that the dwellers in what is commonly called beautiful scenery are often unappreciative of it and indeed more apt to admire scenery of a different kind. Even so I do not think the most

[1]*Republic* III, *Symposium* 210 E.

[2]e.g., Sidney, *The Defence of Poesie* (*An Apologie for Poetrie*). "Even as the childe is often brought to take most wholsom things, by hiding them in such others as have a pleasant tast."

[3]*What is Art?*

[4]Plato is clear that a poem is more dangerous the more poetically beautiful it is. *Rep.* 387, 607, etc.

genuine æsthetic experiences necessarily moralize men. Ruskin[1] says, "Though the absence of the love of nature is not an assured condemnation, its presence is an invariable sign of goodness of heart and justness of moral *perception*, though by no means of moral *practice*; in proportion to the degree in which it is felt, will *probably* be the degree in which all nobleness and beauty of character will also be felt." But I should not think it a relevant testimonial for a position of trust that the candidate was a frequenter of the best concerts and exhibitions, or of Coniston and Chamonix. Nor should I even go to him for moral advice.

§4. We must turn then to the more ambitious theory, corresponding to that of transcendental feeling, which would make æsthetic experience not a propædeutic to morality but a higher or profounder form of it, giving both clearer insight into our duties and a stronger will to perform them.

> In such high hour
> Of visitation from the living God
> Thought was not.[2]

Schiller, as is well known, criticized Kant for distinguishing and even opposing morality and inclination. In the *Letters on the Æsthetic Education of Mankind* he defines the æsthetic experience as the satisfaction of the "play" impulse in a peculiar sense of play as a happy harmony of the sensuous or appetitive impulses with the rational and moral. Thus he seems to hold that the greatest good is not, as Kant held, the fulfilment of duty in the face of difficulty and temptation but "virtue," the lucky coincidence of attraction with duty or what we take to be duty. But in thinking that this coincidence was only or chiefly realized in æsthetic experience he was surely wrong; it might be my pleasant duty in certain circumstances to read poetry or to visit Switzerland, but in others it might be equally pleasant and equally obligatory to lie late in bed or to confer a benefit on one I loved, which I think could not be called æsthetic.

[1] *Modern Painters*, Part IV, xvii, §30.
[2] Wordsworth, *Excursion*, I. 212.

It seems we must conclude that the doctrine of transcendental feeling is correct in its suggestion that what the æsthetic experience signifies is feeling. If by "transcendental" it means that this feeling is always directed to the whole universe or to God or to our duties or that it gives some sort of truth or some cognition better than truth about such objects, I find it hard to understand this and still harder to agree. If all that "transcendental" means[1] is that the æsthetic experience is not a mere feeling like warmth or repletion, but is truly significant of something and makes that something of the greatest interest, this, I think, is true, and we must try to discover in what sense.

§5. I suppose it would be agreed that a beautiful statue or picture need not be exactly like any individual man or landscape, or give us any exact and new information about human anatomy or vegetable or geologic structure, and many would hold that it need not even bear any likeness to natural objects at all, any more than an eastern carpet or cathedral or arabesque need. A beautiful poem need not give us any truthful information of a historical, scientific, or moral or philosophical kind; if it adopts the form of an argument it may be patently fallacious. Some would hold that it need not make any "sense" at all so long as it is a harmonious "significant" string of musical words or even sounds. Yet if it is really significant it must be successfully, that is truly, significant of whatever it attempts to signify. We can hardly resist condemning some alleged works of art as "untrue," "insincere," "affected," "bogus," meaning thereby to give the reason why we think them ugly or failures. Yet we have excluded every kind of truth except the psychological. Is it then that a man has a genuine æsthetic experience when he finds a sensuous image immediately expressive or significant not of his own thinking (for then he would attribute to it scientific, historical, philosophical or moral truth) but of his own feelings, desires, emotions, moods? And is he a successful artist when he succeeds, by fashioning a sensuous object, in communicating this significance to others, whether few or many, who are capable of imaginative sympathy with this mood or

[1] *See* Appendix A.

feeling and therefore can understand what he is expressing?[1]

§6. The expressionist explanation of æsthetic experience is more plausible in the case of poetry than of sculpture and painting, for it was never easy to maintain that the beauty of poetry consisted in its skilful imitation of external realities, but until recently this was a popular theory about the two latter arts. Such a theory overlooked that a Corinthian or Ionic capital is also a work of sculpture, and an arabesque a work of painting. Modern fashion has emphasized that neither painting nor sculpture need be representative, though it has generally maintained that both, like architecture, pottery and embroidery, must, if beautiful, be significant. The only excuse for denying that music is expressive of mental activities, states, moods and passions, is the desire to avoid the error, suggested by "programme music" that what music expresses can be as well or nearly as well expressed in words. But that would be just as erroneous about pictures or statues. Unless we name the notes and describe their sequences and combinations, which might enable a gifted musician to recompose the piece for himself, the best we can say of a musical work is that it is solemn or gay or peaceful or triumphant. That would give more æsthetic information than to call it loud and long or complicated or difficult to execute. And we use similar emotional terms about oriental carpets.

§7. Probably it is natural beauty which seems most repugnant to the theory that all æsthetic experience is the expression of emotions. Yet, if form, colour, movement, sound (and not merely human form or vocal sound) are naturally expressive of such mental states, they might often be found so in nature as well as when artificially exploited. Nothing is more obvious

[1]This is part of the thesis of Croce in his *Estetica* (translated by D. Ainslie, 2nd edition), his *Breviario di Estetica* (translated by the same under the title *Essentials of Æsthetics*) and his article in the 14th edition of *Encyclopædia Britannica* (1929). And *see* Appendix B. It may well be asked why sense should be capable of expressing (as distinct from arousing) feeling. I am afraid I do not know. Kant and Wordsworth in their different ways suggest that it is because our minds and "nature" are "akin." Kant holds that our *satisfaction in* the expressiveness is due to a feeling that the world and our minds are mutually adapted to facilitate perception. But *see* Chapter X.

than that rosebuds express our feelings of or about youth; spring-like colours and sunshine those of cheerfulness; a stormy sea those of fierce or sullen anger. Nobody made them to be expressive, but we, in accordance with our original nature or the second nature of childish and lifelong experience and culture, may find them so as naturally as we do smiles or frowns. A sunset may be as expressive as a chorus-ending from Euripides and a mountain as a Michelangelo. We often do not know whether a child's movements are art or nature, nor æsthetically do we care.

§8. The outcome of such a view, which, with the explanations that I hope to give, I am inclined to accept, would be this: each of us has an æsthetic experience in face of a sensible object (which he then calls beautiful), whether it be perceived, remembered or imagined, when it expresses to him feelings of which by his nature and past history he is capable. His remembrance or imagination may be stimulated by sense impressions not in themselves expressive, such as a printed page or the spoken words "Romeo and Juliet" or "Everest." But just as, owing to his past history, these words might arouse no memories or images, so, owing to his nationality, a printed page of English might arouse none; and owing to his exclusively seventeenth-century culture the sight of Everest might arouse none; and owing to a complete incapacity for sexual passion a love-drama might arouse none (or only by its musical qualities). Consequently there is nothing in itself beautiful; one thing may be expressive to one man, and another to another. But as a great deal of human nature is common to all men, and a good deal to both men and women, and as a good deal of culture is common to all who share a civilization and a great deal to those who share an education, we meet with much actual agreement. Owing to complaisance and æsthetic snobbery we seem to meet with more than we do, for nearly everybody professes to like Shakespeare though very few read him, and not all are so rude as to call our favourite poems rubbish.

§9. Yet we should not expect men and women, black and white, old and young, ancients, moderns and barbarians, Americans and Chinese, classical scholars, rustics and scientists, dwellers in the tropics and the arctic regions, Christians and Moslems, mothers and virgins, Oxford and Cambridge men, to find precisely the same lines, forms, colours, sounds, words expressive in the same way. Mutual contempt is sheer intolerance.[1] Among individuals even of the same family there will be individual differences of organization and temperament; one may be tone-deaf and another myopic, one more sensitive to colour and another to form, they may have varying blood pressures and glands. Each individual too may differ from himself at different times, in health and spirits, in knowledge, opinions and associations, in interest, in memories and in hopes. They have different passions; and all these differences must affect the significance of their various perceptions and images; yet each of these may occasion a keen and genuine æsthetic experience. As Coleridge said, beauty depends on a "shaping spirit of imagination":

> We receive but what we give,
> And in our life alone does Nature live:
> Ours is her wedding garment, ours her shroud!
> And would we aught behold of higher worth,
> Than that inanimate, cold world allowed
> To the poor loveless ever-anxious crowd,
> Ah! from the soul itself must issue forth
> A light, a glory, a fair luminous cloud
> Enveloping the earth—
> And from the soul itself must there be sent
> A sweet and potent voice of its own birth,
> Of all sweet sounds the life and element.[2]

§10. Nothing is lost in the warmth and value of our affections for a mother, a sweetheart, a wife, a daughter, when we reflect that it is only because she is ours that we have this delight in her happiness and virtues, this sorrow in her failures and

[1]Cf. J. R. Sutherland, *Wordsworth and Pope* (British Academy Warton Lecture, 1944). The author points out that Pope confessedly wrote only for the "polite." Wordsworth hoped to be enjoyed by all good men and especially simple men. He has in fact pleased somewhat more widely and probably much more keenly than Pope, and for a time his dogmatism and genius dulled our ears to the niceties of polite expression.

[2]*Dejection.*

defects. It is impossible to believe that those dearest to us are really nearest to perfection. And nothing is diminished in an experience of beauty when we see that, had we been different, we should have discovered it elsewhere and not here. Michelangelo's work was not bad because a Chinaman could hardly have liked it, nor the Chinaman's draughtsmanship because it could hardly have pleased Michelangelo. Both would have had better taste if they could have had more.

Even in morals there is an analogy. The moral experience of self-sacrifice for the good of others is not abated if the results turn out unexpectedly to be for our own advantage rather than theirs; nor, in a converse case, would remorse be diminished by discovering that dishonesty had proved the worse policy. But there is a striking difference here from the æsthetic experience; if we could be convinced that there was not some real duty to others, however hard to know, we should feel no obligation of trying to discover and to perform it, no satisfaction in the effort and no remorse for omission. To deny the objectivity of duty and goodness is moral scepticism; the æsthetic experience is no way abated by the reflection that it depends less upon the nature of objects than upon the significance they have for our interpretation. To assert the objectivity of beauty is æsthetic intolerance; only the denial of real degrees in the purity of æsthetic experience would be æsthetic scepticism. It is purity and vividness we should seek.

CHAPTER IV

FORMAL AND REPRESENTATIVE ART

§1. In past generations æsthetic intolerance generally took the form of insisting upon the importance in art of the "subject matter." Since beauty was assumed to reside in objects, good art would consist in the skilful imitation of objects which possessed it and in the elimination of any defects—in the exact portrayal of the "ideal object." Some men were more beautiful than others; a statue might be more beautiful than any. Some actions were more beautiful than others; the epic or heroic poem or tragedy represented great men doing great actions, perhaps greater than had ever been. Great painting was religious, historic, ideal painting—"the grand style"; *genre* and landscape were inferior; arabesque nowhere.

§2. To-day æsthetic intolerance is apt to assert the irrelevance or positive deleteriousness of any representational element in æsthetic experience, especially in painting but also in sculpture and even poetry. It may be admitted that the pleasure of recognition[1]—that this smudge is just like a fog I have seen or like some old man's face or just like another smudge—would be not æsthetic but an impurity in an æsthetic experience. Yet if sunsets are beautiful, that is to say significant, it is hard to see why the artist should puritanically abstain from employing such significance on occasion. He might aspire to outdo any one sunset just as he might hope to surpass the rendering of light by Vermeer or Rembrandt, the line of Botticelli or the depth of Cézanne. He might even think he could best achieve pure expression of his mood by avoiding the intrusive associations of any natural objects. If this is his belief and this his object it is hard to see why (to cite pictures I have seen) he should introduce into a picture otherwise composed of unrepresentative line and colour patterns a human eye at the end of a proboscis, or a realistic penny bun or

[1]Aristotle, *Poetics, IV*

cigarette; for surely these must have disturbing associations which on his theory are unæsthetic and which are associations with objects less likely in nature to stimulate æsthetic experience than a face, a flower or a bird. Some painters and sculptors refrain from such concessions and produce purely unrepresentative arabesques of line and colour or mass. I am not sure whether they would claim for their works superiority to the best Chinese carpets and vases or the best Greek and Gothic architecture. If they would not, we may ask them why they do not turn their attention to architecture and weaving. If they would, is it because they think unrepresentative art must be small? Similarly when writers like Gertrude Stein produced rigmaroles of more or less euphonious language on the plea of avoiding the unæsthetic associations of subject matter, it is hard to see why they often introduced real words and syntax into the rigmarole, since these have associations, though surely less satisfying than they would have in an intelligible context.[1] If on the other hand they do not use any real words but only unmeaning arrangements of vowels and consonants, we must ask if they would claim to get from these works a keener and purer æsthetic experience than from Beethoven or Mozart. If they would not, we must ask why they do not practise music.

In other words there seems to many of us to be a high empirical probability, not yet invalidated by any exceptions, that there are certain materials and certain magnitudes "suitable" to certain methods, suitable in the sense that they are generally apt to be expressive of feeling and apt to communicate the expression. We may think, for instance, that the purely formal though expressive beauty of a great work of architecture is unlikely to be achieved by a very small unrepresentative object; or that the unmeaning sounds of the speaking voice, however carefully arranged, can never rival song or concerted instrumental music. On the other hand we may think that a human bust as large as St. Peter's would scarcelybe an æsthetic success.

§3. Nobody would wish to veto such experiments, however sceptical he may be of their fortune. If the experimenters claim that they have already succeeded, that geometrical arabesques, perhaps with the help of the penny bun, do give

[1]Cf. R. L. Stevenson's gibe about "opulent oratundos."

them vivid æsthetic experiences more pure than Michelangelo's Medici Tombs or Chardin's still-life in the National Gallery or the earliest Chinese bronzes, we must, if we have no reason to the contrary, accept their good faith. And we shall expect them to be as civil to us. Our thesis, after all, is that beauty does not reside in the sensible objects but depends on their significance and that they must signify something somewhat different for different people, possibly very different for very different people. Perhaps it is no stranger that some people should get a more pure æsthetic experience from a pen-pattern of circles and triangles and others from a Constable, than that Hindoo women should have got the pure moral experience of doing a painful act because they thought it their duty (as we must suppose they sometimes did) in the performance of suttee, and yet should have been unable to get one in incurring unpopularity by slaughtering an agonized cow.

§4. If some of us have any quarrel with the fashionable practitioners of unrepresentative sculpture, painting and verse it is not over the theoretical principle that arabesque and pottery and ἄιλινον, ἄιλινον or "Fol de Riddle Ido" or "Waly, Waly" may have some æsthetic significance, but over the empirical fact that we personally find little in certain rather gat-toothed geometrical designs placed before us. And this is not really a quarrel among those of us who hold that what is called beauty is in fact the significance which certain sensuous forms have for persons of a certain type of temperament and culture. We should really quarrel with those who maintained that the Parthenon "Theseus," or Vermeer's Scullery-maid or Homer's Andromache could not possibly give us a pure æsthetic experience because they had a human significance. That would be sheer intolerant dogmatism.[1] And it would be hardly less so if they maintained that no part of our purely æsthetic pleasure in Botticelli's National Gallery tondo can be due to a life-long familiarity with the Gospels.

[1]K. E. Gilbert, in *The Journal of Æsthetics and Art Criticism*, September, 1947, quotes Malevich (*The Non-objective World*): "In my desperate struggle to free art from the ballast of the objective world I fled to the form of the square, and exhibited a picture which was nothing more or less than a black square on a white background." But why this desperate struggle?

What indeed is wrong with illustration? Only that its appeal may be narrower; it may be all the more vivid so long as it illustrates something that is in our blood, so long as it is to us a natural expression and not a conventional symbol. I see no reason to excuse my own æsthetic experience before Botticelli's Madonna to those who have never had an æsthetic experience in reading the Gospels. Even the undoubted fact that a work of art which depends upon representation can only appeal to those acquainted with the original does not necessarily narrow its appeal. All human beings are acquainted with the human face and form and with some human passions. And some moods or passions are perfectly expressed to some people in painting or sculpture, some in rhythmical language, some in music. It may be that the same or other passions are expressed to other people only or best in irregular arabesques of colour, shape or sound. To me some of Chardin's pictures would greatly lose in sheer æsthetic significance if either the formal pattern were altered or the reference to bread, water, wine and the like objects of universal human significance were eliminated.[1]

§5. Kant,[2] following Hutcheson and Alison, distinguished free or absolute beauty (which he instanced in nature by water-ripples and shells, and in art by arabesques) from dependent or relative beauty, which he instanced by organic bodies (presupposing, as he thought, conceptions of perfection or fitness) and by representative art. Yet he thought both kinds were expressive or significant. Formal beauty expressed to us a certain satisfaction in the harmonious adaptation of our sense data to our faculty for combining them, by imagination and understanding, into objects, as perceptible unities or patterns.

§6. It is noticeable that, concurrently with the unrepresentative mode in painting and sculpture much furthered by Picasso's later style, an opposite movement has appeared in the literature of both prose and poetry. The rhythm or metre so carefully studied for its expressiveness by Tennyson and

[1] I am inclined to put this rather less dogmatically after looking at a painting of luxury fruits and drinks by Monet. But it does not wear so well. *See* Chapter XII.

[2] *The Critique of Judgment*, Part I, 16, translated by Bernard and also by Meredith.

Swinburne, by Ruskin and Pater, the formal plot and point and antithesis elaborated by Meredith and Wilde have given place, in poets of the Eliot school and in prose writers like Joyce and Virginia Woolf[1] to a purely imitative and episodic chronicle sometimes called *rapportage*. In the best writers of this sort, like the last named, this is not the physical realism of Zola, sometimes relevant to the emotions of the characters, sometimes not, but rather an attempt to follow exactly the undirected, almost unnoticed flux of ideas, velleities and images which pass through our minds, however accidental and ephemeral. It may therefore be considered as, after all, expressive of human emotion by representation. It has at least "significance" if not "form." A curious poem by Charles Elton,[2] probably written near the end of the last century, unites the formal and representational tendencies rather differently. "Sense" is sacrificed in some measure to a sound-pattern of inept or unmeaning words, but the purpose, as with Poe, is to gain an emotional and even sentimentally romantic effect. The best passages are put by Virginia Woolf into the mouth of one of her characters in *To the Lighthouse:*

> I wonder if it seems to you,
> Luriana, Lurilee,
> That all the lives we ever lived
> And all the lives to be
> Are full of trees and changing leaves,
> Luriana, Lurilee.
>
> How long since you and I went out,
> Luriana, Lurilee,
> To see the kings go riding by
> Over lawn and daisy lea
> With their palm-leaves and cedar sheaves,
> Luriana, Lurilee.

[1]I should add Proust and perhaps Duhamel if I felt more confident of my competence to judge a foreign style. Virginia Woolf and Proust are probably prejudiced by a sceptical theory, due to Hume, as to personal identity. The above is of course not the only or invariable characteristic of the writers mentioned.

[2]Published in *Another World than This*, an anthology by V. Sackville West and Harold Nicolson.

CHAPTER V

KINDS OF BEAUTY

§1. Clearly underlying the discussion in the last chapter there is a more fundamental problem as to kinds of beauty. There are several conceivable alternatives:

(*a*) The term beauty or æsthetic experience might be used ambiguously. Our experiences in face of an arabesque and of a tragedy might really have nothing whatever in common except that they were both experiences, and this they would also share with experiences which we do not call æsthetic such as feeling sick or eating a steak. This I think may be dismissed.

(*b*) There might be two or more kinds of æsthetic experience which differed in some recognizable character though they also had the recognizable common character of being æsthetic; in other words they would be species of a genus, much as scalene triangles differ from isosceles triangles, though both are triangles. If there were two such kinds one might be æsthetically superior to the other.

(*c*) There might be no distinct kinds of æsthetic experience, though an infinite number of such experiences more or less closely resembling one another; much as there are an infinite number of sizes nearer or farther from one another but no distinguishable kinds of size; in other words æsthetic experience would be an *infima species* of the *genus* experience.

§2. The hankering after distinguishable kinds of beauty has haunted æsthetics perpetually but has never been permanently satisfied. It is noteworthy that in the earliest known æsthetic this quest appears as the distinction between formal and representative beauty developed by Plato,[1] and to be reformulated, as we have seen, by Kant. Aristotle expressed the same thought by saying that poetry is born of two human instincts, that for imitation and that for rhythm, and he also

[1]*Republic*, III; *Timæus* 47; *Philebus* 51.

distinguished two kinds of poet, the man of refined sensibility, taste or fancy, and the man of inspired madness or imagination. "Longinus"[1] distinguished mere beauty or "correctness of style" from sublimity or the "utterance of passion," but prophetically, and perhaps correctly, he blurred the distinction by pointing out that nothing is so fitted for the latter purpose as rhythm. Longinus was rather crudely followed by Burke[2] who greatly influenced Kant's[3] fundamental opposition of the two kinds. Schopenhauer,[4] again perhaps justifiably, shifted the demarcations. He distinguished musical beauty from all other kinds on the ground that it alone expressed the general and fundamental nature of "the Will," that is of the life-force, desire and feeling, while the other arts and nature represented "the Ideas", that is, the various phenomenal manifestations of that "Will" which was the primary metaphysical reality and the cause of all things. Nietzsche[5] followed Schopenhauer's main doctrine but with another shuffle. He held that the "Apolline" or representative arts dealt with the illusory world of separate individualities and, by its beauty, reconciled us to the conflicts and sufferings of that world. The "Dionysiac" arts of music and pure lyric, on the other hand, revealed to us in a mystical and shuddering ecstasy the fundamental basis of individual existence the life-force or will to live. This has obvious affinities with the doctrine of "transcendental feeling."[6]

Hegel[7] distinguished three species of beauty: (*a*) symbolic beauty, the main characteristic of Oriental and pre-Hellenic art, most completely represented in architecture; (*b*) classical art, most completely represented in Greek sculpture, and (*c*) romantic art, represented in music, painting and poetry, perhaps most completely in the last. These, according to Hegel, are different ways, in an ascending scale of adequacy, for

[1]*On the Sublime*, xxxv, xxxix, etc. (translation by Roberts).
[2]*On the Sublime and Beautiful.*
[3]*Critique of Judgment*, 23, etc.
[4]*The World as Will and Idea*, III (translated, Kemp and Haldane).
[5]*The Birth of Tragedy.*
[6]*See* Appendix A.
[7]*Æsthetic* translated by Osmaston. The introduction, which summarizes the theory, is I think, better translated by Bosanquet, and this translation is quoted in the appendix to his *History of Æsthetics.*

representing or expressing the ultimate truth or spiritual reality in sensuous form, though it can only be completely expressed in the non-sensuous form of philosophy. The primitive conceptions of this truth are so vague that they can hardly be expressed at all, or only vaguely by some confessedly inadequate symbol, as when a savage might feel "This mountain or this huge pyramid embodies whatever is eternal and immutable." But in human bodies the Greeks found not mere hints of spirituality but its literal embodiment, its home and natural expression. Christianity, with pagan philosophy, recalled to men's minds that the spirit was after all more than the flesh which embodied it, and that its full nature could not be expressed in limbs however graceful or smiles however sweet. So romantic art is the struggle to express the ineffable by hints, suggestions, shocks; sometimes by wilful crudities and disharmonies. It thus resembles symbolic art but at a higher level. Such was Hegel's view.

§3. The mutual inconsistency of these attempts and their cross-divisions throw some suspicion on the belief that there is any essential distinction to be discovered. And the proliferation of further subdivisions such as the Picturesque,[1] the Grotesque,[2] the Strange,[3] the Dynamic Sublime, the Mathematical Sublime,[4] Typical (or Ideal) and Characteristic Representation (equated severally with the Grand Style and Genre),[5] may look like a *reductio ad absurdum*.[6] The best title to being a distinct species of æsthetic experience seems to me that of Comedy—the grotesque or humorous or ludicrous.[7]

[1]Uvedale Price, *The Picturesque*, and W. Gilpin, *Picturesque Beauty*, and cf. Hussey, *The Picturesque*.

[2]Payne Knight, *Principles of Taste*, I. v. 19 and II. ii. 15–27, 79. Cf. Bergson, *Laughter*, iii. 1.

[3]Peacock, *Headlong Hall*, iv. "Pray, sir, by what name do you distinguish the character of unexpectedness when a person walks round the grounds for the second time?"

[4]Kant, *Critique of Judgment*, 25–8.

[5]Reynolds, *Lectures*, iii; Alison, *Principles of Taste*, iv. 2; Ruskin, *Modern Painters*, XIV, §4; Bosanquet, *History of Æsthetic*, i. Cf. Winckelmann, *Kunst des Alterthums*, IV. ii.

[6]Croce, *Breviary of Æsthetics*, criticizes all such distinctions.

[7]*See* my *Theory of Beauty*, appendix to second and subsequent editions, and cf. Bergson, op. cit.

But it is in some theoretical defences of modern unrepresentative art that the development of such distinctions comes full circle by a return to the original one of Plato. That distinction is between quasi-geometrical or highly stylized or symbolical art and the more emotional, naturalistic, vital art of classical and renaissance times. It is suggested that the creators of abstract, "archaic" or archaistic art had "an entirely different aim in view" from that of the naturalistic schools. Hulme[1] maintains that, in periods when an optimistic philosophy or an unreflective confidence in life prevailed, it was natural to find beauty in an objectification or expression of men's own activity and vitality. "The worth of a line or form then consists in the value of the life which it contains for us. Putting the matter more simply we may say that in this art there is always a feeling for, and pleasure in, the forms and movements to be found in nature." "While a naturalistic art is the result of a happy pantheistic relation between man and the outside world, the tendency to abstraction, on the contrary, occurs in races whose attitude to the outside world is the exact contrary." "Primitive peoples live in a world whose lack of order and seeming arbitrariness must inspire them with a certain fear." "In art this state of mind results in a desire to create a certain abstract geometrical shape, which, being durable and permanent, shall be a refuge from the flux and impermanence." But for the Oriental mind, the author goes on, this fear of the world and alienation from it is not dispelled by advancing knowledge. Their sense of an unfathomable and terrible reality is deeper than that of ancient Greece or modern Europe. Their art remains abstract, but its abstraction is not always satisfied with the production of inorganic forms; it puts man into some geometrical shape which "lifts him out of the perishable world into eternity."[2] This for Hulme marks the Byzantine art, whose essence is austerity and rigidity, as opposed to humanism, which looks on life and finds it good.

[1]*Speculations*. He cites Worringer, *Abstraktion und Einfühlung*, and cf. Riegl, *Stilfragen* and *Spätrömische Kunst-Industrie* and Wölfflin, *Kunstgeschichtliche Grundbegriffe*.

[2]More than the "idealism" of Greek sculpture?

D

This is all consistent with Fry,[1] who says that when formal rhythm is combined with natural appearances, above all with the appearance of the human body, we find its effect infinitely heightened as for instance in Michelangelo's "Jeremiah." Richards agrees: "It may be freely granted that there are great pictures in which nothing is represented, and great pictures in which what is represented is trivial and may be disregarded. It is equally certain that there are great pictures in which the contribution to the whole response made through representation is not less than that made more directly through form and colour. . . . There is no reason why representative and formal factors should conflict, but much reason why they should co-operate."[2] Clive Bell takes the more extreme puritanical view: "The representative element in a work of art may or may not be harmful; always it is irrelevant."[3]

§4. With the principle of all these remarks except the last we have agreed. The beauty we ascribe to sensible objects is really their expressiveness of some feeling—of fear, of confidence, of joy in life, of longing for death, a sense for "the delightful commerce of the world" or for its pettiness and evanescence. But the bisection is artificial. There are not two attitudes to the world but a million, with every variety of bitterness and sweetness: curiosity, longing, languor, rebellion, hatred, despair, trust in God, religious fear, cheerful materialism. And every nation, every age, every individual knows them all. It is absurd to suggest that Homer and the Greek tragedians had little sense of an inscrutable and intolerable fate or that Michelangelo found life a bed of rose leaves. Nor is Hindoo or Chinese art wholly ascetic. Hindoo art is less geometrical than the art of the confident, relatively unphilosophical and optimistic Moslem conquerors.[4]

§5. The impossibility of assigning any really successful work of art, or, speaking more accurately, any notable æsthetic

[1]*Vision and Design*, ii.

[2]*Principles of Literary Criticism*, xviii.

[3]*Art*, i. Also on this question cf. Frances B. Blanshard, *Retreat from Likeness in the Theory of Painting* (New York, King's Crown Press).

[4]*See* Appendix C.

experience, to any one of these alleged species, as well as their cross-distinction, suggests that they are not genuine species at all. They seem rather to be names for elements which go to make up the æsthetic experience, elements which must therefore always coexist in it, whose perfect balance constitutes its perfection, while the undue preponderance of either is a defect. To call a work very classical or romantic, formal or formless, illustrative or meaningless, is generally censure or at least faint praise, except when these terms are used in defence of a theory rather than in direct appreciation. So far as I used the words in praise, I could say no poet seems to me more romantic than Homer or Æschylus or Virgil or Lucretius, no statues than the Parthenon pediments,[1] no painting than the back of the girl with flowers from Pompeii; no paintings more classical than those of Constable[2] or Vermeer, no sculpture than that of Luca della Robbia, no poetry than that of Shakespeare's sonnets; but I could easily reverse the epithets. Nor do I know which to call Milton or Sophocles or Michelangelo or Piero dei Franceschi. When, however, I use either label with emphasis and irreversibly I intend some shortcoming from perfection, however magnificent the aim and sympathetic the achievement: as when I might say that on the whole Botticelli or El Greco or Blake or Rodin or Emily Brontë is romantic and on the whole Raphael or Mino da Fiesole or Pope or Horace or Jane Austen classical. Others would no doubt reverse these reluctant qualifications of devotion, the very utterance of some of which seems blasphemous. That may be due to both or either of two facts which I do not question; either because the terms themselves are shifting and comparative or because different persons must have different æsthetic experiences in face of the same sensible object. And

[1]An obvious exception might seem those of Michelangelo. But the horses' heads in the pediments are more "romantic" than the seated figures in the Medici tombs or the David. The three headless female figures were once actually identified as clouds.

[2]Though, rather unexpectedly, some paintings of Turner's middle period, such as the "Chichester Canal," might be called less romantic than Constable because they achieve their high emotional expressiveness more by a subtle patterning of nature than by impartial imitation.

all this is equally true of natural beauties and of unrepresentative art. Is the Certosa of Pavia or Mozart or Chartres or the Florentine Duomo classical or romantic? Which is Mont Blanc?

§6. If my analysis of æsthetic experience as the expression of emotion is correct it would be natural that on either side of perfect instances, and separated from them by infinite gradations, there should fall instances where passion had been either too strong to attain tranquil contemplation, or so faint as to evaporate in the preoccupation with technique. At one extreme lies mere turbid crudeness and at the other slick or frigid "artistry." But this distinction demands fuller treatment.[1]

I am inclined to think that what lies behind the frequent censure of artists for having "only aimed at beauty" (which surely in strictness should be their only aim) is the meaning that, though sensitive to the beauty already achieved by others and ambitious to emulate it, they have not been impelled or able to originate the expression of their own passions, as their models had, and so remain imitators or "minor poets," without inspiration if not without some charm. They are "silver," facile, polished, finished, versifiers of occasions, practitioners of the grand style, of the *beau idéal* or of *genre*; academic, and, when we soon get tired of them, mediocre.

§7. Most of these attempts to specify beauty could be applied to nature as well as to art, though this has not been so often attempted. All the guide books characterize some scenery as romantic, though perhaps what they would contrast it with would be "pastoral" or "smiling" rather than classical. The contrast between ideal form and individual character is kept up in that between regular human features and expression or charm. "Picturesque" was obviously applied first to nature living or inanimate, though afterwards transferred to its representation. Kant thought sublimity was only to be found in nature, though he gave inconsistent examples. The one distinction that seems confined to art is that of representative and unrepresentative. The nearest analogue in nature might be the distinction between sheerly grand scenery, striking for

[1]For the distinction between classical and romantic *see* Chapter XIV and Appendix D.

its shape, sizes, colour, and that loved for its human associations. Ruskin has noted the difference. In *Modern Painters* he said: "The noblest scenes of the earth can be seen and known but by few; it is not intended that man should live always in the midst of them; he injures them by his presence" (II. iii. 1 §1), but in later life he wrote that the scenery which could most permanently satisfy him was, like that to be seen from Brantwood, enriched by human labour and nourishing human life.

If then we are bent on classifying our æsthetic experiences, perhaps the most fundamental difference is between those stimulated by what we take to be nature and those which we take to be occasioned by the art of other men. Within the realm of art there is the old and useful but not very interesting enumeration of "the arts": architecture, sculpture, painting, music, poetry and "the minor arts." Not only is it difficult to draw the lines but the distinction does not seem to go deep. Some poetry appeals to our pictorial imagination, some to our musical; if sculpture is non-representative it only differs from architecture in size and uselessness. More fundamental might be the senses on which the expressive perceptions or images depend—mainly the eye or ear; we might further subdivide artistic creators according as they mainly express themselves in colours, lines or mass and in melody, rhythm or harmony. But here again poetry is a hybrid. If read it is presented primarily to the eye, or for the blind, to touch, but even so it stimulates the imagination of its sound, and if recited appeals to the ear directly. In any case it arouses images of every sensation external and internal—colour, scent, temperature, pain or pleasure, effort and relaxation. A friend born blind tells me how difficult he finds it to write poetry without using traditional poetic words of which he does not really know the meaning, such as brilliant or dim, and how difficult to use a word such as "distant" to mean only what it means to him, namely a longish journey off, instead of also what it mostly means for us, namely small-looking and hazy. On the whole, classifications of beauty, though convenient for purposes of reference, have shed no light on the nature of the beauties classified.

§8. Finally, we might resign the attempt to classify the arts into kinds and content ourselves with differentiating them in degree of complexity. The most rudimentary would be those which use purely unrepresentative methods, as unsuggestive of natural objects as any perceptions can be: arrangements of colour, line and mass or space, or of sound, though sound must surely have some analogy with the human voice. Next would come representative painting and sculpture, in which the thing represented counts, as Roger Fry claimed, at least as much as the pattern. Literature makes a great advance in complexity. It uses rhythmic pattern and representation, but its representation is not direct but imaginative and can not only present movement, action, and states of mind, but can raise visual pictures almost as vivid as the painter's or sculptor's, as well as tastes, the smell of flowers and the feel of the wind:

"All the charms of all the Muses often flowering in a *single line*."[1]

Our theatre combines literary recitation with gesture, which is an element of dancing, and with painting. Colour can be combined with sculpture, and both with architecture; music can be combined with poetry in song and opera; how far such combinations are successful may be questioned. Ballet may combine only dancing and music or both with literature, of which it then becomes a moving illustration; accordingly it may be either formal or representative.

§9. The most complicated of all arts would appear to be that of the film, which apparently may employ almost every other. Perhaps for this reason its capacities would appear as great as its present awkward age is slow and ungainly. Its future is hard to forecast. Uncertain of itself, it has specialized in the illustration of bad or good fiction, seldom with valuable results, in crude melodrama and childish extravagances. But it ought to be able to outdo both drama and fiction in psychological expression. Once the convention has become familiar, the presentation of a person's fancies, memories, and hopes

[1]Adapted, in the italicized parts, from Tennyson's *To Virgil.* e.g. Κυμάτων ἀνήριθμον γέλασμα and "Brightness falls from the air," and "Murmurs and scents of the infinite sea."

upon the screen is a much better device than the soliloquy or "aside." The "close-up" should be as capable of great uses as of its present abuse. But I think there have not yet been many first-rate works of art on the film, and a student of æsthetics should shun prophecy.

§10. In general, the main purpose, or at least the main result of artistic classification has been the discovery of artistic rules. If every "kind," tragedy, painting, architecture, can be essentially defined as having its proper "end" or idea, then it is hoped that maxims can be devised for the appropriate means—the unities or the universal, the avoidance of illustration or of all reference to nature, or realistic imitation, or truth to material. But these recipes often fail and something else succeeds; there is no recipe for genius.[1]

[1]Cf. G. Boas in *The Journal of Æsthetics and Art Criticism*, June, 1947, p. 208.

CHAPTER VI

EXPRESSION

§1. There here falls to be attempted some elucidation of what has been meant by expression. The repugnance for the term has been due to the confusion of expression with three other things: symptom or sign, symbol, and stimulus or argument.

The "black spot" is, I suppose, a sign of revenge, as a falling glass is of rain. Sweating is a sign or symptom of pain but would not be called its expression, not only because it may be the sign of other states, but rather because we may not know or may only have learnt by hearsay or from one or two observations that it is a sign of pain. The two terms are not for our imagination merged or coalescent but apprehended distinctly, whereas in a smile or frown we say we *see* or feel a man's friendliness or anger and indeed its nature. So a smile or frown, when we are not preoccupied with other matters or with its consequence and the practical conduct it may demand, has a rudimentary æsthetic expressiveness.

It follows clearly from what has been said that another man's expression may be a mere sign for me and give me no æsthetic experience or be expressive of a different feeling. If by some nervous disorder both his parents, and consequently his brothers and sisters, had always frowned with pleasure he might, as an artist or poet, deal with the human face in ways to me baffling.

Perhaps even a single experience, if sufficiently poignant, may make some sensible appearance expressive for one individual though not for another or only in a different way. To Whymper, after his great triumph and great tragedy, the Matterhorn could never have looked again as it may to a hotel guest on the Gornergrat; the last words used by his friends before their fall may never again have had quite the same significance for him nor the same as they have for us.

§2. Even more expressive of human feelings than human faces is the human voice in its timbre, its pitch, its accent, and above all in its language. If a smile or sob is a symptom grown expressive, articulate speech is a symbol that has suffered the same change. From whatever primitive origins language grew it has a conventional or symbolic element. Some words and phrases we spontaneously imitated, some were explained to us by our parents and their meaning "corrected" by our schoolmasters, others we have looked out in the dictionary. For most of us in a foreign language and for nearly all of us in a dead language the conventional element is great. It is chiefly the symptoms and symbols unequivocally significant from our nursery days that become æsthetically expressive of feeling. "Inkhorn-terms," technical terms, terms of art, neologisms, slang not yet naturalized, are notoriously recalcitrant to poetry. Even the valuable use of archaic or learned words to express feelings of strangeness or respect or remoteness, as when we speak of steeds or halcyons or Excalibur, is notably dangerous. Too much "amaranth" is frigid, one nenuphar is apt to suggest Wardour Street; "allergic" and "O.K." are prosaic. But what chiefly makes language expressive is that touch of genius, not wholly lacking perhaps to any man who is capable both of deep feeling and of reflection, which deviates, if only by intonation, alike from mere groans or growls and from the stereotyped formulas of rage or sorrow, into expression. Then we have some degree of beauty. Such a touch of genius in some men may be a feeling for language, in others a sense of form or colour, in others a gift for music.

§3. In distinguishing expression from symptom we have already indicated how it must also be differentiated from symbol. If symptoms may be called purely physical signs, symbols could be defined as arbitrary or intellectual signs. Black is a gloomy colour; why it naturally expresses sadness to us we may not know. Perhaps the optical effect of it may be lowering; perhaps it is intimately associated with winter, night, thunderstorms and ungenial circumstance. Possibly to a negro in a climate where sunlight was a constant peril its associations might be happy, but to us it can in most contexts be *expressive* of sorrow, where it is not obviously conventional as in "mourning." On the other hand scutcheons, flags at half-mast, reversed arms, the removal of shoes or hat, are conventional signs of which any stranger must ask the meaning just as he must ask the meaning of "alas" or "*eheu*" or "*weh*" if he speaks another language. Pure symbols can be translated but pure expressions cannot. When once I have been told that in Greek a semicolon mark has the same significance as a modern note of interrogation I can use it and understand it as precisely as an Athenian, but it may be impossible for me to translate even by a periphrasis the exact expressiveness which "*pietas*" or "*schwärmen*" or "home" have for those who used these words in their nursery. Dürer's woodcut of Melancholy contains a number of curious objects which seem to contribute nothing to the impressiveness of the general design. We ask why they are there and are told they are symbols of melancholy; possibly to some few of his contemporaries they may have become naturally expressive, but for us they have no more æsthetic value than would the title "atrabilious" on the frame. In Rembrandt's etching of the "Three Trees" we find no such symbolic elements but more of significance.

§4. It remains to distinguish the expression of feelings from their stimulation. I might stimulate pity in a man by taking him to a "chamber of horrors" or a hospital, lust by administering a drug, by showing him pornographic pictures or by more direct provocation, but none of these would be expressive of emotion. No doubt to some men the Melian Venus or the Throne of Aphrodite might be sheer pornography, and this is the justification, under certain conditions, of censorship. The dilemma is this: for a creature otherwise human but utterly incapable of any sexual passion no love lyric could as such have any more expressiveness or beauty than music for a man stone deaf; on the other hand for a normal man, not æsthetically disposed, it may sometimes be impossible to consider the expression in tranquillity. Yet for most of us it is possible to see the sculptures mentioned or to read Sappho and Catullus without physical excitement. It is clear that in proportion as feelings are "purely physical" and overmastering, like agonizing pain, untempered by any "sentiment" or "emotion," they are very difficult for the artist to express; perhaps in extreme cases impossible. They are apt to "make our flesh creep," that is to say, to be stimulants rather than expressions; and the same is true of a "purely physical" pleasure, say the eating of a pine-apple, whose attempted expression might merely "make our mouths water." Even if this were not the result to himself of the artist's expression, it would almost certainly be the result of the attempt to communicate it.

§5. For lastly the expression has to be distinguished from its communication, which is not—like symptom, symbol, stimulus—something exclusive of it, but something that can be done to it, though also to other things. I can communicate the significance of a symptom or a symbol by explaining it, and a desire by the stimulus of drugs, example or realistic suggestion. I find it difficult to say in other words how I communicate an æsthetic experience, that is to say the expressiveness which some sensuous image has for myself, to another person. I am inclined to use the word "infection."[1] I fancy that most artists somewhat modify their internal image by emphasizing or understating some details in order to concentrate the recipient's attention rightly, to avoid probable misleading associations or expectations, and the like; just as in speaking to a foreigner in our own language we should use a more staccato articulation than was natural since, if we did not do so, we might communicate nothing more expressive than nonsense noises.

§6. Under the communication of stimulus we must class propaganda and indeed argument. This is the attempt to induce beliefs or feelings, which may probably result in actions, by appeals either to the emotions or to the intellect. The reliance on symbols in a work of art is merely a confession of æsthetic weakness, but the intermixture of edification, incitement or didactics is a sin against the æsthetic spirit. Nothing is so poisonous to the purity of an æsthetic experience as the feeling that an artist has palpable designs upon us. At once the question of historical fact or of moral truth is raised:

[1]If this metaphor suggests stimulus, I could only substitute 'rouse an echo.'

Did our enemies really behave so vilely? Was our side really so pure-minded? Ought we really to behave in this way? Is there not also much to be said upon the other side? If such questions do not disturb us, it is because the orator has flattered our passions and we mistake a hymn of hate for a poem about hatred. The tranquil contemplation of expressed passion is troubled by these storms; sympathy cannot flourish in political meetings. And on the other hand confessed propaganda is weakened for the critical mind by any reliance on pseudo-lyrical or rhetorical assaults upon our emotions. We do not want as jurors or as legislators or even as philosophers to be charmed or thrilled by pictures but to be convinced by well-documented facts and hard logic. Uplift is neither art nor argument but a hybrid, unfortunately not sterile.[1]

§7. The artist's intention here is something we need not inquire into. Like Scott or Trollope he may have sat at his desk for money, like Dickens, sometimes, to remedy abuses, or, like William Morris, sometimes, to enlist us in a political cause. But so far as they were men of genius or inspiration, their pens were guided by the spirit, and what we can read is pure expression of suffering, pity or indignation. Whether a man who lived when their subject-matter was one of burning controversy could have read them as we do does not matter. We cannot help feeling that what we read must have been sheer beauty, not argument, to the writers; we know it is to us. Perhaps if a man could have read *Rob Roy* in 1715 or 1745 he would have wanted to ask questions and to argue. Perhaps a contemporary of Dickens would have inquired into the evidence about Poor Law administration and chancery procedure, as we feel compelled to-day to ask for the facts behind the tendentious pro-and-con novels of the Near East. As it is we can see in the picture of Rob Roy or Oliver Twist or Tite Barnacle the expression of something truly human, something we might ourselves be or do or suffer. It may be that to Pontius Pilate a picture of the crucifixion must have appeared tendentious, an attempt to win approval for an anarchical movement. To a Christian (and for these purposes all modern men are

[1]Cf. Chapter VIII. 'Rhetoric' sometimes denotes 'prose poetry', sometimes propaganda.

Christians) it may appear a pure expression of voluntary suffering, innocent and without resentment.

§8. It remains then to distinguish the expression of emotion from the communication of that expression. This is difficult, for the word expression is usually employed to denote expression to another person, and there is no other single word in our language to denote, what surely occurs, expression to oneself. I am said to express my feelings in a poem or sonata and it is assumed that this must be written, perhaps printed, published or performed and sold, and indeed read or heard and understood. But surely my æsthetic experience on the completion of the poem cannot be altered by the accidents of the bookselling trade; nor even by the sensibility or obtuseness of other people. It was expressive to me and may or may not be expressive to other people. I think it in accordance with ordinary usage, that is proper usage, to confine the term "work of art" to some externalization in the way of utterance or other sound, writing, gesture, painting or plastic art, which is capable of stimulating a somewhat similar expressive experience in others. But I may compose a quatrain or a melody in my head and keep it there and it will be none the worse for that; if I were a foreigner in China it would be no good doing anything else with it. And if it cannot then be called a "work of art" it can perhaps be called an artistic creation or invention.

§9. Another reason for this confusion between expression and communication is the fact that few people can create artistically on a large scale without externalization. However it may have been when writing was unknown, to-day few men can compose an epic[1] or an opera without pen and paper, or at least an instrument, though Mozart seems to have been an exception. And in painting and sculpture the imaginative memory is still more narrowly confined.

This leads us to the distinction between art, in the sense of artistic creation, and craft or technique. A great composer might be a poor executant, and before writing was invented a great poet who was a poor reciter would have been no better

[1]Travellers in illiterate countries still tell us of poems several thousand lines long recited with verbal accuracy though never written. Perhaps the authors composed them aloud though alone.

off. The distinction is usually drawn that whereas the mere craftsman works to a pattern or specification, or at least to solve a precise problem, such as how to carry water of a certain volume to a certain spot, the creative artist does not know how his creation will turn out till it is completed but then sometimes sees that it is good. He may know that he wants to express a feeling, but till he has expressed it to himself he only feels it, he does not, so to speak, appreciate or discriminate it; he is troubled or exhilarated as an animal or child may be; he is like the awakened dreamer who can often only tell that his dream was horrible or gracious or somehow oblique, but not *what* it was. The line is hard to draw, for something of the same kind seems true of the solution to a new problem in pure mathematics or geometry. Yet it remains a fact that artistic creation discovers its aim only, if ever, in the achievement, which may or may not require the aid of some material upon which to experiment and record, such as paper, wax, a pipe or a piano. But once this internal expression has been perfected, its communication, however difficult or impossible, would be a matter of craft; we should know already what it is required to do. So then for the production of what is commonly called a "great work of art" two distinguishable qualities seem required, though we may think it probable that they usually coincide: imagination or inspiration and craft or technique, a distinction which has sometimes also been misleadingly indicated by the opposition of genius to taste. A man of great imagination may remain mute or inglorious, a man of exquisite technique may remain a mere imitator, or, worse still, an originator of uninspired works. The distinction may be illustrated from a poem which I greatly admire, number XXIII of A. E. Housman's *More Poems:*

Crossing alone the nighted ferry
  With the one coin for fee,
Whom, on the wharf of Lethe waiting,
  Count you to find? Not me.

The brisk fond lackey to fetch and carry,
  The true, sick-hearted slave,
Expect him not in the just city
  And free land of the grave.

This might fail to convey an æsthetic experience of the writer for two reasons. The reader might not have the classical education enabling him to understand the allusions of Lethe and "the one coin." This is no defect in the work of art, but, if anywhere, in the tower of Babel and in our social system. No poem can be addressed to readers who speak a different language or have a different culture. But even to the best classical scholars there is an obscurity in the first stanza which cumbers the effect. Does it mean "When you are crossing the ferry, whom do you count to find waiting on the wharf?" or "When you are waiting on the wharf whom do you count to find crossing?"? On careful re-reading surely the former. But the need for careful re-reading owing to an ambiguity in syntax is a defect distracting us from perfect enjoyment. Not, however, I think, a defect in the poetic vision of the author who, I presume, noticed no ambiguity—or he would have corrected it—and therefore was not distracted. It is a defect of technique or handicraft.[1]

[1]If I had been quicker-witted I might have jumped to the correct meaning without hesitation; but that does not affect my argument. Cf. Shakespeare (*Winter's Tale* IV iii) "Daffodils that——take the winds of March with beauty," where *take* may mean 'receive' (e.g. the sail takes the wind) or 'captivate' (e.g. B. Jonson *Silent Woman* I.; 'Such sweet neglect more taketh me'). And see below XIII §3 note on Arnold.

CHAPTER VII

EMOTION

§1. Having endeavoured to elucidate the first term in the phrase "expression of emotion"—expression—we must turn our attention to the second—emotion. In the first attempt we distinguished "expression," as here used, from symbol, symptom, infection and communication. In the following we must try to meet two opposite criticisms: first that of those who urge that our definition is too wide since not all emotions can be beautifully expressed, and second that of those who urge that it is too narrow since beauty, natural or artificial, may be expressive of other mental states and activities than emotion. (A) The first objection, that the expression of some emotions cannot be beautiful, may rest on two grounds.

§2 (i). It may be, in a general sense, an ethical argument. It is held that some emotions are so bestial, monstrous or wicked that their expression can only be vile. But the question is: are they human emotions at all and does the expression enable us to find them human; are they emotions with which we can "sympathize" in the sense of feeling that in other circumstances we could have felt them? If so, our moral condemnation of acting from such passions, or of encouraging them, does not condemn our æsthetic satisfaction in thus coming to realize their nature. When a villain's emotions of envy, hatred and malice are thus expressed we can but say, "I am a man of like passions," while hoping that we may never be of like actions and praying to be delivered from temptation.

When the artist goes further and, in his own person or through the mouth of his characters, pretends to glorify cruelty and injustice, without motive or temptation, for their own sakes, we feel that this is not the expression of any human experience, as when Richard III says, "I am determined to prove a villain." Iago also comes near being a mere stage figure.[1] On the whole his satanism is attributed by others, as

[1]See Ch. XI.

the expression of their own disgust, rather than self-claimed unless in half-ironical bravado. The villainy of Edmund, too, however vile, comes near being intelligible as a revolt against the injustice of fate. Milton has clearly struggled, and only with partial success, to reconcile the theological necessity of keeping Satan devilish and the æsthetic need of making him credible. Macbeth and his wife are far more human, though not less criminal, than Richard and Iago.

The presentation of untempted saintliness is almost as difficult; probably no passage in the Gospels has been so touchingly felt as the prayer for the removal of the cup.

Yet in consistency with the doctrine of the subjectivity of beauty outlined above, it must be remembered that what was successful expression to the artist may not be so to some of his audience whose experience has been different. When, however, satanic or divine boasts are made in the artist's own person we are bound to think them a pose imposing on nobody but himself.

§3 (ii). The second argument to show that not all emotions can be beautifully expressed is more considerable and is to be considered on psychological rather than ethical grounds. Can vomiting, cramp, the taste of *pâté-de-foie-gras*, any mere pang or titillation, be expressed æsthetically? The obvious answer is that these are not emotions. That word was chosen rather than "feelings," since the latter generally covers mere sensations. The problem may not seriously arise for most of us in the instances just given, but it does when we are confronted with "tales of horror," "shockers," and "thrillers," whether graphic, linguistic or in any form which makes our flesh creep. In descriptions of purely physical ecstacy or anguish what is described may more properly be called a "commotion" than an emotion, and is perhaps incapable of expression. If we again take Wordsworth for our guide, poetry must be emotion recollected in tranquillity. We may remember that we had a moment of pure bodily torture, but if we really call up again the quality of the experience as well as the temporal fact we can hardly remain tranquil; we can believe that others are in agony, but if we indeed realize their sufferings we are ourselves physically affected. Illustrations of torture on the one hand or of the sexual act on the other have in general, and for ordinary spectators, no æsthetic appeal: the better paintings of the crucifixion stress the mental rather than the physical torment. Emotions are feelings which have risen or been raised from the status of sensations to what we may call a higher level, higher not morally but in the sense that they presuppose the "lower" and are not presupposed by them; we are often apt to think that they are only possible for beings rational as well as sensuous, and it may be observed that we also think only such beings capable of æsthetic expression.

The distinction here drawn between sensation and emotion is nearly parallel to that often made between pleasure and happiness (or pain and misery). Happiness, it is said, requires self-consciousness, a sense of identity in time, which pleasure does not. I suppose that even on the way to the stake I should *feel* the pleasant sensation of eating a peach, as the sinner just assured of salvation feels the toothache, but since neither of us would attend or contemplate, the emotional tone of neither would be much affected.

So far, the instances taken of "commotions" have been sensations more or less localized in the body, but I think we must class with them "mental" states which are organically disturbing, such as panic terror, "seeing red," and all animal motions which are more infectious than expressible. Euripides in the *Bacchæ* attempted the expression of some, but perhaps has only succeeded in perfectly communicating his expression to those of like genius. What must remain mere commotions in most men and in the lower animals may be capable of rising to emotions in a highly intellectual sensibility by the mere fact that such a one is able to contemplate them and so to give them rudimentary expression. This might be what led Croce to assert the identity of intuition, if by that he meant contemplation, with expression. Emotion is not sensation but sentiment directed to an object, in Croce's language a movement of attraction or repulsion.

§4 (B). It remains to consider the converse objection to our definition of æsthetic experience as the expression of emotion. This objection is that the expression of other activities or states besides emotions may be beautiful. We have already remarked that a mathematical argument may be expressed perfectly, that is to say, clearly and tersely, without giving us the distinctively æsthetic experience; and something similar may be said of the illustrative diagram or of a working model in a physical laboratory. More crucial instances are in the didactic poem or the expression of historical opinions, and these will be treated in the next chapter. At present it may be granted that no intellectual activity is unaccompanied by some feeling—of weariness, curiosity, exhilaration, ease or impediment. And, as was hinted in the last section, only when, under some physical duress, we lose the human in the animal, are we capable of sensation unmodified by the work of mind. But it remains true that, as a doctor may distinguish his scientific interest in the case from his humane interest in its cure, though the two are in fact for him inseparable, so we can distinguish between our factual or logical interest in a book and our concern in that communication of the writer's "personality" which can hardly ever be quite absent. This is perhaps most noticeable when we read history or argument in a foreign language, and especially in a dead one, or in an archaic idiom; for here words intended to be colourless have for us an impressiveness of their own. The multiplication table is however the limiting case, where a meaning is expressed in any language without noticeable emotion.

CHAPTER VIII

DIDACTIC AND PROTREPTIC ART[1]

§1. In the last chapter an objection to the definition of beauty as the expression of emotion was cited to the effect that art, and perhaps nature, may be beautiful through the expression of other mental states and activities. In distinguishing emotions from sensations I have implied that the latter are not æsthetically expressible. The remaining faculties traditionally recognized are thought and will. It has been granted that no concrete experience of a sane human mind can consist of any one of these in pure abstraction from the others. It remains to ask whether in an æsthetic experience we may be predominantly concerned with the expression of the intellectual or conative element of the whole activity expressed, or always with the emotional.

(A) I will deal first with the intellect.

§2 How charming is divine philosophy!
Not harsh and crabbed, as dull fools suppose,
But musical as is Apollo's lute,
And a perpetual feast of nectar'd sweets
Where no crude surfeit reigns.[2]

How surprising the epithets and assertions seem to-day! But they have not only dramatic propriety in the mouth of the rather naïve second brother; they were commonplaces of contemporary criticism. In 1607 Jonson wrote "Doctrine is the principall end of Poesy, to inform men in the best reason of living."[3] Spenser was as often praised for his philosophy and high morality as for his sweet "numbers" and "invention."

It is clear that much great poetry could only have been

[1]On the subject of this chapter I am much indebted to conversations with my pupil, Mr. J. Hartland-Swann, who is preparing a work on philosophical poetry.

[2]Milton, *Comus.*

[3]*Epistle Dedicatory to Volpone.*

written by men of speculative powers: Lucretius, Dante, Milton are names which spring to mind; Wordsworth claimed a philosophy and, in a loose sense, was justified. And the great majority of poets, like the great majority of men, show some interest in ethical, historical and political questions, some in the existence and character of a god or gods, nearly all in sexual passion. And on all these topics they have differed and even contradicted one another or themselves. Dante's philosophy is incompatible with Lucretius. The tragedies and comedies of Shakespeare reveal very different views about life and love. If then a man enjoys alike Dante, Lucretius and Milton, *As You Like It* and *Troilus and Cressida,* it is hard to suppose that such enjoyment depends upon the nature of the philosophy or the theology or the moral opinion expressed; it must depend upon something common to them all. This cannot be the fact that *some* theory or other is being expressed for that would be common to Aristotle and Kant and Mr. Richard Turner[1] who are not considered poets. It must then depend either upon something unconnected with the theory, such as metrical skill, metaphor, simile and the like (these, too, it has been argued are expressive, and surely not of doctrine) or upon the expression of emotions occasioned by the belief held, not upon the belief itself. And this seems to be the truth. Most of us have had our moods of scepticism and our moments of faith, or at least of hope; and those of us who have had both can appreciate both the expression by Lucretius of his delightful triumph in escape from superstitious terror to clear thinking and also the expression by Dante of his consolation in divine love and justice. True philosophy and false can alike occasion poetry if they have moved the poet; so can the reading of history or falling in love or the loss of a friend.

I do not claim that the seventeenth-century critics believed this. Few men to-day distinguish clearly between the satisfactions they receive from knowledge, from moral worth and from beauty. In a less analytic age, especially one fascinated by a somewhat uncritical reading of Plato and the Platonists, the confusion was inevitable.

When in a later time Keats said that beauty is truth and

[1]To whom we owe the term "teetotalism."

truth beauty, I am not sure what he meant, but I think he was not subject to the same confusion. Perhaps he meant that poetry must be true expression of real feelings; perhaps that the æsthetic experience is real and important. If he intended it in any more usual sense of truth it is hard to see how he would have squared it with the other passage that "fancy cannot cheat so well. As she is fam'd to do," where the fancy spoken of is his own poetry.

§3 (B). The confusion just noticed in the seventeenth century between æsthetic satisfaction and the satisfaction of finding one's own beliefs and ideals ably expressed persists in many minds to-day. Perhaps most people demand that poetry should have "a message," by which they generally mean a "directive" to political action either by rational argument or more often by emotional appeal; and the direction must, of course, be one in which they are inclined to go. In this they are somewhat excused by the poets themselves, who often make a merit of toeing the party or religious line. Such poetry may more properly be called protreptic (or vulgarly "mob-poetry") than didactic, since it deals little in historical or economic facts but much in sarcasm and slogans. Lord Baldwin, who had a scholarly sense, once said that rhetoric was the harlot of the arts. He was thinking mainly of its loose uses in politics, but in poetry it is no less venal.

The implied theory then must be that æsthetic expression is the expression of the conative or willing element in any concrete experience, the expression not of a mood the poet has felt, but of a policy on which he has acted, and of a policy moreover which the reader must himself embrace if the æsthetic experience is to be communicated to him. The logical conclusion would be a censorship by the majority on grounds of political orthodoxy, a device obviously consistent with totalitarianism and tempting to all of us so long as we believe we are in a majority; when we know we are outnumbered it is a conclusion we do not draw. Plato envisaged such a censorship by the omniscient rulers of his ideal state, but he did not make the blunder of thinking that their decisions would be on æsthetic grounds. The argument against this protreptic theory is similar to that previously used against the didactic.

If we can equally appreciate a Puritan and a Cavalier marching song our appreciation cannot depend on the nature of the willing expressed, but only on something common to both. This again cannot be the fact that *some* willing or other is expressed, for that is common to most election speeches and also to "Rule Britannia," which has been more effective than Blake's *Jerusalem*. But it might depend on the fact that in each item was expressed a genuine enthusiasm. Even this conclusion however will not quite meet the conative theory we are now discussing. Macaulay's *Epitaph of a Cavalier* ("To my true King") cannot have expressed a conviction on which the writer was prepared to act, but only a mood he could imagine and sympathize with in others. Nor do I suppose that either Heine or Schumann in their words and setting of *Die beiden Grenadiere* were Bonapartists except in imagination.

It is precisely the imagination which "will-theories" of æsthetic expression leave out.

If "conation" or similar words are used, as by Croce, in a wider sense to cover not actual willing only but all "movements of attraction or repulsion" this would bring us back to emotion as that which in the æsthetic experience is expressed and in the work of art communicated.

§4. My instances have been taken from poetry because this seems most favourable to the didactic and propagandist theories I have been criticizing. It would be harder to maintain that painting (except posters), music and architecture express or communicate beliefs or policies. It seems likely that they do this for emotions, which may arise either from the beliefs really held and policies really willed or from others merely entertained by the imagination. And the purely æsthetic experience of those to whom the expression is communicated presupposes only a similar entertainment.

There is, however, a fashion even among contemporary painters for what may be called serious caricature, analogous to the savage satire of the Roman Empire and some of our Augustans. Imitating Goya and Daumier, though seldom with their power or skill, they invent ghastly parodies of the human face and figure, intended no doubt to express their indignation at men's vice and folly, but which either afford most of us a sour and sorry amusement or madden us with their crudely vindictive temper.

§5. Adherents of the propagandist theory are apt to sneer at the purely æsthetic experience of art and nature as "escapism" or "an ivory tower." No doubt it is an escape both from the rare atmosphere of pure thinking and from the brazen Babel of party strife, which in turn is an escape from pure thinking and from the vision of the tragic artist, as pure thinking is an escape from all the rest. The only censurable escape is from one's duty, which in different situations may be by turns artistic, intellectual or political. Perpetual confinement is the fate of the monomaniac.

John Stuart Mill once asked himself how men would employ their ample leisure when the utilitarian Utopia had been attained, and answered that he hoped they would read poetry and enjoy nature. Perhaps the hope was rash; at least, if in the meantime men neglected all but propagandist art, it would be disappointed. We work and fight to get peace and ease for the enjoyment of thought and beauty and our affections, and perhaps also to play; though no doubt our thought and our affections themselves will always afford new objects for our efforts.[1]

[1]The didactic fallacy, from which primitive men, when they distinguished art from magic, were comparatively free, was imposed by Plato and has now seeped into the lowest strata. An old villager, fond of reading, lately lamented to a friend of mine that, through 'lack of education,' he had missed much pleasure in that way. He was introduced to *Oliver Twist* and expressed keen delight, only qualified by the disappointment that 'though I'm told that to read Dickens is an education, there's none of that here. I just seem to be living in it all.' I find this rather pathetic.

CHAPTER IX

THE TASKS OF CRITICISM

§1. If the view of art here put forward is accepted, what must be the function and value of criticism? Under that name are loosely comprised two purposes essentially different though generally combined and sometimes overlapping. The first is that of establishing and interpreting what may be called the actual text or artefact of the artist. This, as we have said, is properly a branch of history. And if by history be understood not so much a record of dates, governments, conquests and economic changes as a sympathetic understanding of the thoughts and feelings of men in past ages, then no branch of history is more significant than such artistic criticism. For, as a great historian has confessed, it is works of art which are the best key to men's hearts: "Between us and the old English there is a gulf of mystery which the prose of the historian will never adequately bridge. They cannot come to us, and our imagination can but feebly penetrate to them. Only among the aisles of our cathedrals, only as we gaze upon their silent figures sleeping on their tombs, some faint conceptions float before us of what these men were when they were alive."[1] I have myself never had so strong an impression of insight into an alien religious enthusiasm as in the gloom of the tiny but grimly ponderous chancel of the Norman Church at Leuchars near St. Andrew's. And if this is true of architecture and sculpture it must be even more so of mosaic, of painting and of poetry.

§2. It is clear that some of this art-scholarship is very far removed from æsthetic valuation though some comes very near. At one end of the scale are the excavators, the restorers, the papyrologists, the grammarians, the picture cleaners who enable us to recover and piece together the debris of the past. Their work need be no more æsthetic than that of the men who

[1] J. A. Froude, *History of England.*

first discovered for the civilized world the Grand Canyon or the azalea. Then come the textual critics and the learned commentators who explain the allusions, the manners and beliefs of the times, the shades of meaning and literary association in the syntax, the words used or the scenes depicted. For the best work in this kind almost the same sensibility and taste are required as for criticism in the more precise sense, and it is here that the borderline between the two is often crossed. Ruskin for Gothic times and Pater for the Renaissance have not only explained what the artists may have meant but greatly helped us to enjoy them, and this last Ruskin has also done for many aspects of nature. Arnold has enlarged and refined our sympathies by his distinction of "Pagan and Medieval Religious Sentiment."

§3. From what has been already said about the subjective character of beauty, it might seem that this is the only function of the critic—to widen our æsthetic appreciation—and that therefore he is improperly called a critic or judge, being in fact only a writer of testimonials. But really he is concerned as much with purifying as with extending our æsthetic experiences. It will be perfectly proper for him to suggest that many professed admirers of Milton's poetry have been mainly occupied with his theology or his politics, and that perhaps Milton himself was sometimes so distraught. Dickens was often, we must suppose, more anxious to exhibit poetic justice and to paint abuses in the blackest colour than to portray truly the working of men's or children's hearts. The critic can divert our interest from these defects to the really expressive elements in great writers.

§4. Indeed we might be inclined to think that the critic's only capacity for extending our æsthetic appreciation was that of a pointer or anthologist. And it is true that he treats the work of art somewhat as the original artist is apt to treat nature, emphasizing what is of interest, clearing the sky or shrouding the insignificant in haze. What more, it may be asked, could he do? Is not even such emendation a censure of the work he is criticizing? "If water chokes you, how will you wash it down?" If you know the artist's language and his allusions and if he is a good artist, but cannot communicate to you his message, are you not incurable unless by a long education or a deeper experience of life? Yet the fact remains that there is something more which critics can do for us. They can somehow put us in the mood. If I were minded to obstruct a man's appreciation of a work of art I think I should know how to set about it. Aristotle advised the rhetorician to meet his adversary's lofty appeals with ridicule and his ridicule with seriousness. So I should decry genuine pathos as sob-stuff and tragedy as highfalutin; I should immunize against *Epipsychidion* by the sober realities of everyday life and against Crabbe by the platitude that we do not live on bread alone. The critic's true task is the converse of this, though I cannot reduce his talent to a rule-of-thumb. Certainly the whole significance of a work of art cannot be exhausted in any medium but its own, but since we are all more conversant with the art of language than with any other, a man to whom sculpture or architecture or music has been a closed book may be introduced to it by the words of one who has himself enjoyed it. Something of the same kind is attempted for literature by illustration, though naturally with less success except when addressed to the illiterate. What the critic can do for literature, especially of an unaccustomed kind, as for the other arts, is to put us in the right mood, to tune us to the artist's pitch; he can, as it were, transpose this alien music into a more familiar mode. It is at any rate indisputable that Ruskin, for instance, influenced both taste and practice in architecture and painting, whether for the better or the worse, as well as the taste for nature; and if it is possible to influence, it must be possible to influence for good.

§5. Ruskin was himself a draughtsman, especially of mountain, sky and architecture, and a colourist of some merit, and it may be that the criticisms addressed severally to artists and to their public should be different in kind and are different in their effects. Criticism of poetry seems naturally to come from literary men who pursue a similar art. Painters and musicians and architects may reasonably ask whether they too do not deserve to be criticized only by their peers, that is to say not in literature but by someone with a brush or instrument or model in his hands, carrying on, as it were, the work of a teacher or *maestro*.[1] It cannot be doubted that practitioners of all the arts are influenced by criticism, in their own practice as well as in their appreciation, often very narrow, of schools and periods different from their own. They have generally had a teacher and would surely claim that they are never too old to learn. Imagination, that is the creative part of art, may be stimulated, and the technique of communicating the image can, like any other craft, be taught to those who have the knack.

[1]Cf. *Free House or the Artist as Craftsman*, by W. R. Sickert, ed. O. Sitwell. Turner seems to have thought that the best criticism of a picture by Claude was to hang one of his own beside it.

CHAPTER X

THE GENESIS OF ÆSTHETIC EXPRESSIONS

§1. The way in which various sensuous presentations—colours, sounds, lines, shapes and objects—have become specially apt for æsthetic significance must get its explanation from physiology, and especially neurology, from biology, psychology, and especially child-psychology, from anthropology and the general history of culture. Clearly no student of any one of these sciences can give an informed opinion on the conclusions of the others, and nobody can be competent in them all. Consequently most of the work remains to be done; perhaps the most serious attempt has been that of the psycho-physiological schools of *Einfühlung* or "Empathy" (inward sympathetic imitation) headed by Lipps in Germany and ably discussed by Mitchell in *Structure and Growth of the Mind*.

§2 (i). It seems established that some colours and sounds are *physically* stimulating and others depressing to our nervous system and occasion changes in pulse or breathing. These, especially when organized in patterns, might naturally become expressive of the exhilaration, melancholy, or other moods which they have occasioned. The nerves of eye and ear may be more apt for exuberant exercise because more recuperative from fatigue. It is possible that certain lines or shapes might have similar direct physical effects. It was formerly maintained that a curve is more agreeable than a jagged line because the eye followed it more easily in one continuous sweep, but eye-photography now seems to have proved that in perceiving a curve the eye moves with short rectilinear jerks.

§3 (ii). (*a*) *Psychologists* have offered several suggestions of ways in which perceptions may have acquired æsthetic significance. The most respectable, at least by its antiquity, is an elaboration of Aristotle's *Unity in Variety*. Kant held that, in distinguishing individual objects from the blur of sensations simultaneously presented to us, our minds generally unify the "manifold of sense images" under some concept of the understanding. It is easy to pick out a man or a house from the surrounding landscape, unless they are artfully camouflaged; it is easy to distinguish known words or phrases or the dinner-bell from the flux of sound, and none of this gives us any æsthetic satisfaction. But there are some arrangements of shape and sound, representing no previously known objects, which by their own symmetrical or repetitive character facilitate or compel their apprehension as unities or "patterns"; they "fit together" though we cannot say as what. In these cases Kant holds there is a *free* harmony of the imagination and understanding, as distinct from a *controlled* or practical harmonization in the recognition of familiar objects. This free harmony gives us a peculiar satisfaction, due, as Kant thinks, to an appearance of design but design with no other purpose than to facilitate our apprehension. To this he attributes the beauty of music and arabesque, and of ripples, shells, and the like natural objects. It is worth remark that, so far as our fragmentary monuments go, though palæolithic art was naturalistic, as explained in the next section, geometrical patterns held a dominant place in the art of the following era which presumably was house-building rather than troglodyte.

(*b*) More important, at least historically, is the play theory used psycho-physically by Burke[1] and in less *a priori* fashion by Spencer,[2] and philosophically by Schiller.[3] Burke argued that visible beauty pleases us by relaxing in some way the bodily tension, producing what he calls a pleasing languor; the sublime pleases by terrifying, since it thus gives safe exercise to some "finer parts" of the brain or nervous system which, in normal civilized life, stand in need of exercise and are benefited by what Aristotle called "purgation." The weakness of this explanation as a differentia of sublimity is betrayed by the admission that greater "safe terror" can be derived from the spectacle of a real execution than from any tragedy, and Burke remarks with apparent approval that the audience would always leave the theatre for a hanging. Spencer, returning on empirical grounds to something like the view of Schiller,

[1]*Sublime and Beautiful.*
[2]*Principles of Psychology.*
[3]*Letters on Æsthetical Education.* See above, III §4.

held that æsthetic enjoyment is the "play," as distinct from the life-preserving function, of any faculty or organ; and this occurs among the higher animals, whenever any organ has a superfluous energy which seeks some useless exercise. These uncalled for exertions are most displayed by those organs, like the eye, which take the most prominent part in the creature's life, but unlike the palate, are not closely bound to biological services. Here again it seems clear that the definition is too wide. Much play and voluntary exercise, stretching, jumping, thumb-twiddling, "ragging" can hardly be considered art.

(*c*) More relevant, if less empirically verifiable, psychological suggestions are those of the *Einfühlung*, "Empathy," or "Inward Imitation" school of psychologists, which recall Aristotle's conjecture that one chief factor in the poetic experience is our delight in imitation. They hold that in every concentration of attention upon an individual object within the sensory field, by a kind of unconscious animism, we read into it sensations or emotions of our own. I feel myself as striving, triumphing, yielding, free, cowering, not "over against" the thing but, somehow, "in it." And this is the ground of the satisfaction I take in the object, for the object is my self objectified; the distinction indeed has been obliterated or rather has not yet become clear. Sometimes in watching an athlete's struggles we overtly initiate movements similar to his, more often our motions are merely incipient and internal; in any case the æsthetic experience is quite different from conscious imitation, for it is, so far as we are conscious of it, purely contemplative, and we are not aware of our own limbs or organs. It differs too from the impersonations of deliberate mythology, not only from absurd instances as "Inoculation, Heavenly Maid, descend!" but, as Wordsworth saw, from more imaginative but still conscious fable:

> Brook! whose society the Poet seeks,
> Intent his wasted spirits to renew;
> And whom the curious Painter doth pursue
> Through rocky passes, among flowery creeks,
> And tracks thee dancing down thy water-breaks;
> If wish were mine some type of thee to view,
> *Thee, and not thee thyself*, I would not do

Like Grecian Artists, give thee human cheeks,
Channels for tears; no Naiad should'st thou be—
Have neither limbs, feet, feathers, joints nor hairs:
It seems the Eternal soul is clothed in thee
With purer robes than those of flesh and blood,
And hath bestowed on thee a safer good;
Unwearied joy, and life without its cares.[1]

Elsewhere[2] he regrets the natural impersonation which, before the "world was too much with us," could. . . .

Have sight of Proteus rising from the sea
Or hear old Triton blow his wreathèd horn.

Empathy is also distinguishable, in spite of border-line instances, from mere habitual association of feeling with an object where each is distinguished from the other. At this point the school diverged into two sects, one emphasizing solely muscular feelings such as lifting at sight of a column, springing at sight of an arch, the other laying its main stress upon "emotion," such as conflict, gaiety, gloom, eagerness, fear and the like, which are activities of our "self," not of our "body." An attempt is made to explain the apparent contradiction of "experiencing our own activity in an object" by an analogy with the way in which we re-live our own past experiences as part of ourselves yet not our actual selves. The gist of the theory is that a thing expresses to us the feelings which we know or think that we or other people have who look or move or sound in the same way as the thing. This is true and important. But something more has to be said. Not only may we delight in the running of the deer because it reminds us of our own childish delight in motion, but we delight in waves and cataracts, whose motion we cannot share, because we imagine their feelings if they could feel like us, and this is exactly the opposite of "inward imitation"; it is outward projection. Moreover, our pleasure in this æsthetic fellow-feeling even when the object's supposed experience is unpleasant or vicious, as it is in tragedy and

[1]Sonnets II. xxxi. My italics.
[2]Sonnets I. xxxiii.

pathos, remains unexplained. Lipps is puzzled by our æsthetic pleasure in the trouble and despair of Faust or in "a gesture of foolish vanity." It is significant that these writers generally speak only of "suggested" feelings; Croce offers a more promising formula in "expression," since it is plausible that to become aware of the nature of what we had previously only suffered might be a profound satisfaction. We must return to this in a discussion of æsthetic sympathy.

(*d*) The word "expression" suggests the last psychological doctrine we need consider. Psycho-analysts have asserted that all æsthetic experience and creation is the release or "sublimation" of emotions hitherto repressed and "unconscious" or "subconscious." This too seems to have an Aristotelian origin in the doctrine of "purging the emotions." But unlike Aristotle who instanced pity, fear and religious ecstasy as feelings to be discharged, the moderns have often considered only the sexual instinct. For this no very convincing evidence has been offered and some of the attempted applications to great artists and works of art are discouraging. But that in æsthetic experience we come to a clearer consciousness of our own natures and capacities may be allowed.

§4. (iii) (*a*) Some colours, sounds and objects also have become attractive and in course of time expressive to human beings by *biological* evolution; individuals who attended to them or used them may have profited in longevity and consequently in the power of transmitting their innate sensibility to offspring. Among our animal or remotely human ancestors those who were highly sensitive to the approach of weather changes must have had a far greater chance of survival, and this gift may have developed into a deliberate concentration on clouds and mists, winds and stars. Some of our earliest literary expressions of a love for celestial signs, in Homer and the Old Testament, suggest this process:

ὡς δ' ὅτ' ἐν οὐρανῷ ἄστρα φαεινὴν ἀμφὶ σελήνην
φαίνετ' ἀριπρεπέα, ὅτε τ' ἔπλετο νήνεμος αἰθήρ,
πάντα δὲ εἴδεται ἄστρα, γέγηθε δέ τε φρένα ποιμήν[1]

[1]*Il.* VIII. 555. "Even as when in heaven the stars about the bright moon shine clear to see, when the air is windless, and all the stars are seen, and the shepherd's heart is glad."

and Psalm CIV. The way in which these practically interesting goings-on became expressive is shown first in the creations of mythology, by which men projected their own life and feelings into what excited them, as nymphs and dryads, fauns and satyrs. Later and more conscious stages of the activity are constantly exemplified by Virgil:

> In freta dum fluvii current, dum montibus umbræ
> Lustrabunt convexa, polus dum sidera pascet[1]

and, at a later stage, the poet, having personified nature, uses its assumed feelings to express his own:

> Sidera per viridem redeunt cum pallida mundum
> Inque vicem Phœbe currens atque aureus orbis,
> Luna, tuus tecum est: cur non est et mea mecum?
> Luna, dolor nosti quid sit: miserere dolentis.[2]

As men became hunters, fishermen, shepherds and farmers they had to concentrate their attention and sympathies on the ways of wild and domestic creatures, and on the habits of vegetable growth. It is hard to think that the palæolithic cave-paintings of big game, whatever magical purposes they may also have served, were without æsthetic interest. Early poetry is a constant fancier of the horse in his warlike and peaceful uses. Homer and the author of *Genesis* both loved a garden:

> ἀλλὰ μάλ᾽ αἰεί
> Ζεφυρίη πνείουσα τὰ μὲν φύει, ἄλλα δὲ πέσσει.
> ὄγχνη ἐπ ᾽ ὄγχνῃ γηράσκει, μῆλον δ ᾽ ἐπὶ μήλῳ,
> αὐτὰρ ἐπὶ σταφυλῇ σταφυλή σῦκον δ ᾽ ἔπὶ σύκῳ.[3]

[1]*Aen.* I. 607. "While rivers run into the sea, while shadows move across the mountain slopes, while stars have pasturage in heaven."

[2]Appendix Vergiliana, *Lydia* 39. "When the first faint stars come out over the heaven, still green, thy lover Endymion is with thee, Lady Moon: why is not mine with me? Thou who knowest the pains of love, Lady Moon, take pity on a lover." (The reading of the second line, which I have omitted in translation, is doubtful.)

[3]*Od.* VII 118. "Evermore the west wind blowing brings some fruits to birth and ripens others. Pear upon pear waxes old, and apple on apple, yes and cluster ripens upon cluster of the grape, and fig upon fig.

If grapes gladden man's heart the rose is lovely in itself and adorns the head of the feaster; an "anthology" is a garland of flowers; the rosebud is a natural analogue of youth.

Not even the war-horse who "saith among the trumpets Ha, Ha and smelleth the battle afar off" inspired so much early poetry as the sea, the team of Poseidon, white or "wine-dark," or with its myriad dimples ἀνήριθμον γέλασμα, for from the sea and the stars a sailor can never take his eyes. From the beginning dawn and dusk, stars and dew, birds and deer, fruit, flowers, the sea, and, among the works of men's hands, fire have been the sensuous images which poets and artists have found expressive of their feelings. And the mere catalogue suggests one of the passions they have most commonly been found to express, and therewith an object biologically forced upon mankind's attention even more strongly than the sky and soil and food by which individual life is sustained.

(*b*) The human body is the means by which our strongest appetites are gratified and the race is carried on, by which the tribe is defended, the prey hunted, the fields tilled; every muscle and organ has its significance. And the human face is instinctively read as friendly or hostile, proud or shy, wise or foolish, happy or sad. Not surprisingly have sculptors and painters returned again and again to the "express and admirable form of man" to signify the passions of the lover and the enemy, of the parent, the child and the friend. It is not necessary to be a Freudian to recognize how great a part the universal instincts of sex and parenthood have played in artistic iconography. Unlike the other motives for expression which we have noticed, the sexual interest is bifurcated. The interest of the more domestic sex in the habits of the weather and the game may be less than man's but it is not different. All creatures, not least children, and to a less extent even animals, have a significance somewhat different to women and to men, either because they are babies or because they are of a sex.

(*c*) This differentiation of effects is more or less common also to the *social* influences which now fall to be considered. The bodily structure of most of us, apart from sexual differences, is pretty similar; the psychology of our perception must be even more so; among the ancestors of us all there must have been nomads, shepherds, farmers, sailors. But in their later histories our stocks may have diverged. Not only have they known different climates but not all may have experienced long periods of empire or slavery, of devil-worship or philosophic speculation, of magic or rationalistic culture. Consequently the mythologies of Greece, of China, of India, of Scandinavia, of Palestine differ æsthetically. The chief social influence that need be common to every race is the survival-value of loyalty to the community whatever shape that community has taken. So the eminence in poetical symbolism which is sometimes now ascribed to the Leader-myth or *Führerprincip* must be very variously interpreted for peoples with clannish, feudal, servile or theocratic histories behind them. Similar differences may be expected to arise between monotheistic and polytheistic, polygamous and monogamous, war-worn and sheltered peoples, islanders and mountaineers.

§5 (iv) There remains the most recent differentiation, perhaps less fundamental but more conspicuous by its individuality, depending on *personal* history from the nursery to the university and subsequent vocation. Town-dwellers will tend to use somewhat different æsthetic expressions from those of countrymen, though this may be much modified by literature; brothers and sisters will not speak quite the same language as only children; boarding and day schools have their different tastes as much as the rich and poor; athletes and bookworms, parsons and lawyers, landowners and shop-keepers, farm labourers and factory hands admire diversely. But overriding all these differences is that of education in the wide sense. This is most obvious in literature. A period which was bound to be more generally familiar with the authorized version of the Bible than with any other book could hardly help using a simple but imaginative style; in a parliament where ministers were expected to quote Horace if not Homer a certain felicity of utterance was frequent; Shakespeare has modified the English tongue. In the other arts similar influences can be found. Our architecture was no doubt influenced by the national genius as much as it influenced it, but Vandyck, who set our aristocratic ideal for some generations, was a foreigner. I do not know if it is fanciful to suppose that the acquisition of the Elgin

Marbles by the British Museum, at a time when most of Europe knew little but Roman copies of the Greek, has formed our taste in the human figure and in the plastic arts.

§6 (iv) The extreme degree of individuality in expression must arise from associations of ideas depending not upon the cultural environment or social relations but on sheer *accidents* of personal life—the scenery in which one has been happy, the book one was reading or the music heard when one suffered some great loss, the features and complexion of one's friends. Such an association may give true æsthetic significance to objects if its origin is forgotten or only recalled with effort, so that the sign and its meaning are not thought of separately but fused.

Ruskin, who seems to have invented the term "pathetic fallacy" remarks "the difference between the ordinary, proper and true appearances of things to us and the extraordinary, or false appearances, when we are under the influence of emotion, or contemplative fancy. . . . So long as we see that the *feeling* is true, we pardon, or are even pleased by, the confessed fallacy of sight which it induces; we are even pleased, for instance, with those lines of Kingsley's,

> They rowed her in across the rolling foam—
> The cruel crawling foam

not because they fallaciously describe foam but because they faithfully describe sorrow. But the moment the mind of the speaker becomes cold, that moment every such expression becomes untrue, as being for ever untrue in the external facts. And there is no greater baseness in literature than the habit of using these metaphorical expressions in cold blood."[1] Wordsworth[2] had already said "The poet . . . is a man pleased with his own passions and volitions, and who rejoices more than other men in the spirit of life that is in him, delighting to contemplate similar volitions and passions as manifested in the goings-on of the Universe, and habitually impelled to create them where he does not find them."

[1] *Modern Painters,* IV. xii. §4.
[2] *Preface to Lyrical Ballads.*

§7. The cursory essay of the preceding sections is enough to show that any convincing valuation of the various factors in the growth of æsthetic significance must await the maturity of several embryonic sciences and the industry of some proficient in them all. It has been reported by psychologists that the "most æsthetic types" experimented upon express their appreciation of paintings by emotional words like gay, bold, lively; another type describes the formal pattern; a third mentions private associations with the subject, colour or shapes; a last records personal physical reactions such as shivering or sweating. But it seems question-begging to call one type more æsthetic, and the results await confirmation. In the meantime it is regrettable that an easier though uncongenial way of shedding some initial light on the question has not been much followed. It would be interesting if more people would risk the censure of egoism by a candid confession of their earliest uninspired æsthetic experiences however absurd. Early sand castles and brick buildings are lost in the mists of infancy; it is hard to tell whether the toy animals of babyhood were less or more purely æsthetic than the animal paintings of palæolithic man. The first things I can be pretty sure that I found beautiful without adult or literary suggestion were, at perhaps the age of five or six, a blazing fire and a burst of golden crocuses. Much later, perhaps at about nine or ten, I was seriously puzzled by my parents' enthusiasm over natural landscape. My first recollected experience of tragedy is Hans Andersen's story of the twelve swans. Of my infantile efforts at creation, never communicated, the earliest I remember was an endless saga continued every night in bed, probably based upon Old Testament history, about the deeds of two heroes named Huz and Buz; the next was the drawing of geometrical flower patterns with compasses. I ought to add that I have always had a bad ear. I exclude "pretending," whose origin again is lost in antiquity—being a train, being a bear or a bus-conductor, or a red Indian on a rocking horse. I think many of the alleged childish efforts at pictorial art are rather to be called histrionic—impersonations of "father writing."

§8. Much of what has been suggested in this chapter was clearly indicated by Alison, whose *Essays on the Nature and*

Principles of Taste are undeservedly forgotten, though they would seem to have influenced successors from Kant[1] to Bosanquet. This lack of recognition may justify quotation. "In the human body, particular forms or colours are the signs of particular passions or affections. . . . In such cases, the constant connection between the sign and the thing signified, between the material quality and the quality productive of emotion, renders at last the one expressive to us of the other. . . . There are analogies between silence and tranquillity—between the bustle of morning and the gaiety of hope."

[1]His *Critique of Judgment* was published in the same year (1790).

CHAPTER XI

ART, SYMPATHY AND IMAGINATION

§1. There is an obvious connection between æsthetic experiences and sympathy, but before we can be sure what the connection is we must try to elucidate the vague term. Kant held that the sympathy is only with our fellow-admirers of public beautiful objects, natural or works of art, or at least only arises from a confidence that a private æsthetic experience would, if communicated, be similarly valued by them. This sympathy, as he saw, is strictly extraneous and subsequent to the pure æsthetic experience. It cannot be doubted that we do delight in sharing our æsthetic pleasures as we do those of the table, of knowledge or of gossip, and more deeply. Most of us enjoy discussing with a friend the poetry, novels, music and pictures for which we have a common taste; and we like to have him with us in good scenery. But the question is whether, in some proper sense of the word, sympathy is integral to a private æsthetic experience.

§2. Etymologically sympathy means fellow-feeling. In modern usage it means something akin to love, in fact pity or admiration, the recognition of an experience in others which we not only could feel but should approve or at least not disapprove ourselves for feeling. I may be well able to feel lust, hatred, greed, intolerance, but try to check the overflow of these feelings in myself and have little or no sympathy, in the second sense, with those who do not. To sympathize with his characters in the first and weaker sense is clearly a principal virtue of the dramatic or narrative artist whether in prose or verse; that is only to say he must make them credible as possible human beings, first to himself and, if he communicates, to his audience. Many readers find even such sympathy impossible for sadist or masochist characters or for those who profess a disinterested cult for evil. Dickens, for instance, has, I think, succeeded in giving us this kind of sympathy for Mr. Dombey but not for Carker or Ralph Nickleby. If even this measure of fellow-feeling is unattainable and yet the monstrous character cannot be relinquished, what the artist does is to treat it "extrinsically," to express not how it feels to itself but the loathing or contempt it arouses in some observers. This method is usually applied only to a small minority of the persons in any one work; in satire to all.

In the non-representative arts such as arabesque and music it is clearly impossible to sympathize or make others sympathize in either sense with the subject-matter. Neither the artist nor his audience can imagine what it feels like to be a cube or a fugue, still less approve their feelings. Only so far as he communicates his expression does the artist aim at *arousing* sympathy and then it must be sympathy, in both senses, with himself. He wants his hearers to feel as he does and to feel no repugnance at the feeling, but, for the moment, to abandon themselves to it. And this must also be the aim of every work of fiction; its purpose in making us realize the persons presented is to make us sympathize with the artist's whole vision.

§3. The empathy school, as we have seen, holds that by a fundamental psychological law we have a tendency to imitate, at least internally, all those activities which we perceive in animate things or project into the inanimate. We are infected by the gloom or gaiety of our human and animal neighbours, or as Hume put it, "The minds of all men are similar in their feelings and operations; . . . As in strings equally wound up the motion of one communicates itself to the rest, so all the affections readily pass from one person to another. When I see the *effects* of passion in the voice and gesture of any person, my mind immediately passes from these effects to their causes, and forms such a lively idea of the passion as is presently converted into the passion itself." We have to remember, however, that this mere infection with real or feigned emotion, as distinct from its contemplation, need by no means be æsthetic; there is nothing beautiful in mob-anger nor in the most suggestive pornography or advertisement. We must try to define further.

§4. A word even more constantly used in æsthetic criticism than sympathy is imagination. Indeed, it is offered as the magic key which would unlock all the mysteries of beauty—if only we knew how to turn it. When, for instance, we have heard that Dickens is full of crude melodrama, false pathos, ridiculous sentiment, propaganda and caricature, we are told that it is all brought alive by his imaginative genius. And with the necessary changes the same may be said of *Jane Eyre*. We may agree that life comes but we are little wiser about its origin.

Etymologically, once more, imagination is the faculty, present in all men but differing in degree, of calling up more or less vivid images of sensuous objects or internal states, which are, we believe, all memories or combinations of memories. Some people can almost see in their minds a red light or a friend's face; almost hear the siren or, like Mozart, the symphony, and in abnormal conditions this may pass into illusion. A high ability for this vivid reproduction of past experiences is extremely useful to the artist and probably very conducive to æsthetic experience in general, but it does not seem to be the most essential quality. And I can imagine vividly, say, a fly or a speck of sawdust or sleepiness without æsthetic experience. Even the native ingenuity of combining different images in a new way was distinguished as "fancy" from vital æsthetic genius by Coleridge, who, if he popularized imagination as a "blessed word," at least went so far towards defining it. Wordsworth in his 1815 Preface helps a little more, at least by his examples. As an instance of fancy he cites Shakespeare's description of Queen Mab as

> In shape no bigger than an agate-stone
> On the fore-finger of an alderman.

For imagination he splendidly quotes his own

> Motionless as a cloud the old man stood,
> That heareth not the loud winds when they call,
> And moveth altogether if it move at all.

and Shakespeare's

> I tax not you, ye Elements with unkindness,
> I never gave you kingdoms, call'd you daughters,

and Milton's

> Attended by ten thousand thousand Saints
> He onward came; far off his coming shone.

Shelley in his *Defence of Poetry* is more explicit and says that to "imagine intensely and comprehensively" a man "must put himself in the place of another and of many others; the pains and pleasures of his species must become his own." We see already how nearly the æsthetic uses of "sympathy" and "imagination" coincide. John Stuart Mill in *Poetry and its Varieties* says "Poetry, which is the delineation of the deeper and more secret workings of human emotion, is interesting only to those to whom it recalls what they have felt, or whose imagination it stirs up to conceive what they could feel, or what they might have been able to feel had their outward circumstances been different. . . . The truth of poetry is to paint the human soul truly."

§5. The outcome of these two discussions seems to be that the sympathy and the imagination which are demanded both for æsthetic experience and for communication are really identical. It is again Wordsworth who, in his first *Preface to Lyrical Ballads*, has most clearly seen this to be true for poetry; and it is as applicable to the other arts: "The Poet . . . has a greater *knowledge of human nature*, and a more comprehensive soul, than are supposed to be common among mankind; a man pleased with his own *passions and volitions*, and who rejoices more than other men in the spirit of life that is in him; delighting to *contemplate* similar volitions and passions as manifested in the goings-on of the Universe and habitually impelled to *create* them where he does not find them. To these qualities he has added a disposition to be affected more than other men by absent things as if they were present; an ability for conjuring up in himself passions . . . whence, and from practice, he has acquired a greater readiness and power in *expressing* what he thinks and feels, and especially those thoughts and feelings which . . . arise in him without immediate external excitement. . . . Poetry . . . is the impassioned expression which is in the countenance of all science . . . carrying sensation into the midst of the objects of the science itself. . . . Poetry . . . takes its origin from emotion *recollected in tranquillity.*"

The significant words here are those I have italicized. The stress on contemplation and tranquillity preclude the error, which we saw might be suggested by loose talk of either sympathy or imagination, that in æsthetic experience we actually undergo passions or in the work of art communicate them to others. Here they are imagined passions felt only by "sympathy." At the same time it is emphasized that what is imagined, created, imputed, contemplated and expressed must be passion, and it is the expression of passion which must be communicated. Mere vividness of imagery is assigned its due subordinate part in the artist's equipment, and so is the technique of communication. Perhaps Wordsworth's æsthetic theory is almost as good, in its humbler office, as his poetry.

CHAPTER XII

SELF-CRITICISM (I)

§1. Psychological æstheticians appropriately commend us to the empirical rather than the *a priori* method of substantiating our hypotheses. But here the only data we can directly experience are those of our own minds; reports by other people of theirs are even more apt to be misleading. It might therefore be useful, in substantiating what has been said in the previous chapters, to attempt a candid autobiography of some crucial æsthetic experiences. This is not criticism in the dignified manner as a work of literary art, nor is it aimed at æsthetic propaganda or the justification of personal preferences; it is an apologetic attempt to explain, so far as possible, the ground for such of my tastes as I am persuaded are genuine, in the belief that analogous grounds exist, *mutatis mutandis*, for the different preferences of others. I make no pretence to fine taste but only to strong affections, and my blind spots will be just as instructive as my enthusiasms.

§2. I propose to begin with painting, as on the whole offering the simplest problem. It shares with all non-literary arts the difficulty for this purpose that what it expresses cannot be accurately expressed in words. But on the other hand poetry, fiction and the films are in many ways more complex; architecture is usually on a scale which necessitates perspectives and allows a part to be accepted while others are rejected, at least—as with the proposed restoration of Coventry Cathedral—the interior or the outside; sculpture in the round may also be seen from various points of view. Of music I cannot speak.

I shall therefore first pose several questions which have puzzled me about some of the pictures I have most intensely enjoyed and give such answers as I can.

(*a*) What makes me prefer Vermeer to De Hoogh whose aims often appear similar?

De Hoogh's colouring is generally more arresting and

brilliant, his pieces being usually or always in direct sunlight. But though Vermeer's figure-pictures are, so far as I remember, with perhaps two exceptions, in subdued or interior light, the light, the furnishing and the figures are somehow more intimately fused, expressing a subtler emotion if producing less sensuous exhilaration. It is as if De Hoogh's people just happened to be doing their chores in cheerful weather, while Vermeer's must be reflecting "How delightful to be thus talking, thus playing in this cool, harmonious atmosphere!" They might be saying with Marvell "What wondrous life is this we lead!" (A silver thought in a silver shade.) There is something of the same quiet atmospheric perfection as in Henry James's best novels. The picture which used to be in the Vienna gallery, of a maid peeling potatoes I think, has all this with more than De Hoogh's vitality and brilliance. This cannot be the whole story, since with the exception of the last-mentioned picture I enjoy Vermeer's city landscapes even more than his *genre*. But they have a similar intimacy; they seem painted not by a tourist in search of the picturesque, but by a citizen who has learnt the best hour of daylight for the river-front and the street corner and knows who work and live there.

(*b*) Why does Chardin's still life please me incomparably more than any other?

There is much in the mere pattern of the objects as placed within the frame, seldom rivalled unless perhaps, among moderns, by Sir William Nicholson. There is something, perhaps æsthetic, in the engrossingly realistic technique. But for me I am sure the value of all this lies most in the significance of the objects chosen, in something which would doubtless disappear without the pattern and the technique, but which never comes to birth in paintings, equally realistic, of profuse grapes and peaches, pheasants, and lobsters by Hondecoeter. The homely beauties of black bread and draught wine seem in Chardin's consecrated hands to acquire an æsthetic sacramentalism.

(*c*) Why has Botticelli always been one of my favourite painters?

No doubt the sheer calligraphy counts for much, as in Chinese painting; but the savour of the two is very different. The eastern line breathes sophistication if not disillusionment, sometimes grim, sometimes humorously tolerant, sometimes pathetic. Botticelli seems to me essentially youthful, spring-like, I might say virginal; for surely the Venus and the *Primavera* and the Madonna tondo of the National Gallery, whether passionate or maternal, playful or pensive, are all in the spirit of their spring and golden age.

(*d*) Why am I partially blind to El Greco?

His predominant colour scheme with magentas and mauve shadows, his elongations, his flickering lights and restless draperies, are to me irritant. More serious is the intrusiveness by these means of a religious attitude with which I hardly sympathize, a yearning without the austerity of the Byzantine school, of Piero dei Franceschi, and of Milton or the humane piety of the fifteenth-century Florentines and St. Francis. I come nearest to him in his portraits, as the knight in armour of the Louvre, or in quasi-portraits as the St. Jerome in the Scottish National Gallery; these are like Donne's *Holy Sonnets*. The only point of this confession is that I read and hear eminent art critics praising just those elements in the pictures which alienate me; and they praise them because of their fusion in and expression of a religious attitude with which, owing to their greater catholicity of imagination, they can sympathize, but from which I am shut off.

(*e*) Of less personal predilections less need be said. For the figures of Rembrandt and Velasquez analogous grounds of pleasure hold good as for Vermeer. Rembrandt's virtuosity of glowing gloom on armour or on jewels or books is fused to a harmony with the character portrayed, it is a light in which they live and have their being. The distance and focus of Velasquez put his groups and persons, as it were, in the place where our interest wants them, makes them inhabitants of our intimate world and its "delightful commerce." Apart from the great Rokeby Venus I find his early style on the whole more moving, as in the so-called "Christ in the Home of Mary and Martha," and "The Supper at Emmaus" in the Beit collection. The faces of the cook-maids are more keenly felt than those of the monarchs, their working garments more significant than the velvets which, after all, were designed by court tailors.

In rural landscapes probably the sketches of Constable

have given me most lasting enjoyment, though Monet's best work was at first sight more thrilling. This preference pleases me because I can be pretty sure that Constable enjoyed in his pictures almost precisely what I do. He speaks of the nature which inspired him in the very terms I could myself have wished to find for his works; and of Cozens he says: "He is the greatest genius who ever touched landscapes . . . he is all poetry." This master of technique dedicated it all to the communication of feelings which had been expressed in his vision of trees and clouds.

§3. In sculpture my most vivid experiences have come from the Greeks, especially the Parthenon pediments, from Michelangelo's Medici tombs and from the renaissance monuments of Ilaria del Caretto and Guidarello Guidarelli. These three forms embody to me severally the perfect equilibrium of human nature, its tragic poise in oscillation, and its quiescence. I am wholly blind to modern unrepresentative sculpture, which never has for me the impressiveness of architecture or of the earliest Chinese bronzes. But, again, the interest of this defect is that I have heard enthusiastic eulogists of the unrepresentative give just the reason for their appreciations which I have suggested for mine. I will cite Mr. Clive Bell, though I cannot recall his words except "significance," and will quote a criticism which has been endorsed to me by artist-friends: "By the interpenetrations of the material, the convergence and recession of the planes, the dissolving curves . . . the sculptor is enabled . . . to identify his own emotion not with the wave but with the curve of the wave."[1] Once more, the lesson is that some so-called abstract art is to some minds expressive of feeling, that is to say beautiful, in just the same way in which some representative art is to nearly all. The peculiar affection I have for Luca della Robbia's "Visitation"[2] is also illustrative of this point, if less obviously.

§4. In architecture perhaps the buildings which have most moved me as a whole are the cathedrals of Chartres[3] and

[1]E. H. Ramsden on *The Sculpture of Barbara Hepworth* in *Polemic*, September—October, 1946.

[2]Before the late war in S. Giovanni Fuorcivitas at Pistoia.

[3]Its expressiveness is well described by Pater in *Gaston de Latour*.

Tarragona; of interiors St. Mark's at Venice, though this may be called rather mosaic than architecture, the chancel in the Norman church at Leuchars, near St. Andrews;[1] of exteriors Wells and Salisbury, the domes of the Radcliffe Camera at Oxford, of St. Paul's and of the cathedral at Florence, and the west front of Durham seen from Prebends' Bridge. The last undoubtedly owes much to its situation, and this is interesting as showing the indistinguishable contributions of art and nature to beauty. Among less complex wholes or features the chapter house steps at Wells[2] and Magdalen Tower at Oxford, especially as seen from the round in the Botanic Gardens,[3] would rank high; cloisters, Jacobean manor-houses and Lombard churches would be favourites. Two façades specially endeared to me by close familiarity are the east end of the Oxford Cathedral, as altered by Sir Gilbert Scott, and the meadows-front of Corpus Christi, both visible from the same spot as Magdalen Tower.

It is relevant to my main theme that architecture is to me one of the most emotional arts and yet the most "abstract" one which appeals to me strongly. I have had great pleasure from Greek architecture, but, I now think, partly owing to its literary and historical associations.

[1]Again Pater has found the apt words: "Religions . . . grow intense and shrill in the clefts of human life, where the spirit is narrow and confined."

[2]"Sure so light a foot
Did n'er wear out the everlasting stone."
Romeo and Juliet.

[3]Of which Pope said that it was not only like a picture but like a picture hung. (Spence.)

CHAPTER XIII

SELF-CRITICISM (II)

§1 (D) Since literature is the only art which, in common with all who can write, I practise, the application to it of what I have said about criticism, imagination and sympathy should deserve a separate chapter. And in the department of literature the seniority of poetry will hardly be questioned.

In the galaxy of poets it would be of less interest for my purpose to join a chorus of homage for the few fixed stars than to essay the grounds of my affection for one or two particular planets, who naturally enough are among those familiar to my youth. It is really only one's own tastes on which argument can be surely based. Why, I may ask myself, among the Victorian luminaries, do Matthew Arnold and Swinburne please me more deeply, if less often, than Tennyson or Browning?

I propose to trace in Arnold the various elements of imagination I have suggested, beginning with the simplest and going on to their complex fusion in the greater passages.

Arnold has been popularly damned, and even rather faintly praised by Saintsbury, as a highbrow poet, pessimistic, colourless, didactic, dull. My reasons for liking him are that I find him simple, sensuous, passionate. But his passion is certainly remembered in tranquillity; his sensuousness is less copious than Swinburne's but never so crude as that can be. Yet the passion is not so often forgotten in the tranquillity as it is in the virtuosity of Tennyson. His simplicity contrasts strongly with Browning's weakness for the intellectually involved and bizarre. It may therefore be that Arnold has a natural appeal to the student.

§2. The most elementary form of "imagination," predisposing and necessary to poetry, but not by itself achieving great things, was said to be the faculty for forming vivid images, either simply reproduced or compounded from separate experiences. The Keats who wrote *The Eve of St. Agnes* would, I think, have been pleased with:

Happy he who lodges there
With silken raiment, store of rice,
And for this drought, all kinds of fruit,
Grape-syrup, squares of coloured ice.

I have a fretted brick-work tomb
Upon a hill on the right hand,
Hard by a close of apricots
Upon the road of Samarcand.

The very excess of detail here is a sign of poetic power, youthfully exuberant, not yet harnessed. It is used with rarer atmosphere in:

And on the conjuring Lapps he bent his gaze
Whom antler'd reindeer pull over the snow;
And on the Finns, the gentlest of mankind,
Fair men, who live in holes under the ground.

Sometimes this fertility of imagery runs over into a Whitman-like catalogue:

A flute note from the woods,
Sunset over the sea!
Seed-time and harvest,
The reapers in the corn,
The vine-dresser in his vineyard,
The village-girl at her wheel!

but it soon gets bent to better purpose:

For very young he seem'd, tenderly rear'd;
Like some young cypress, tall and dark and straight,
Which in a queen's secluded garden throws
Its slight dark shadow on the moonlit turf
By midnight to a bubbling fountain's sound.

or in:

While the deep-burnish'd foliage overhead
Splinter'd the silver arrows of the moon.

where the vivid image expresses our own surprise at familiar objects seen in a strange brightness; and in:

As a spray of honeysuckle flowers
Brushes across a tired traveller's face
Who shuffles through the deep dew-moistened dust
On a May evening in the darken'd lanes.

where it is our sudden awakening from dull routine that surprises. Then comes the set simile where the image is no longer a charming toy to be quickly dropped, but a sensuous picture of the feeling it illustrates.

as a cunning workman in Pekin
Pricks with vermilion some clear porcelain vase,
An emperor's gift—at early morn he paints,
And all day long, and, when night comes the lamp
Lights up his studious forehead and thin hands.[1]

This is a miniature poem in itself, an experience we may all know but expressed in an alien picture. If it seems a little frigid or decorative in the poem where it occurs, another, no less individually sympathetic, is perfectly congruous with the whole theme:

As some rich woman, on a winter's morn
Eyes through her silken curtains the poor drudge
Who with numb blacken'd fingers makes her fire—
At cock-crow on a star-lit winter's morn
When the frost flowers the whiten'd window-panes—
And wonders how she lives and what the thoughts
Of that poor drudge may be.[2]

But more imaginative than any simile is the unconfessed metaphor where the poet seems hardly to know if he is talking

[1] *Sohrab and Rustum.*
[2] Ibid.

of nature or of his own mind and the minds of men:

Thin, thin the pleasant human noises grow,
    And faint the city gleams;
Rare the lone pastoral huts—marvel not thou!
The solemn peaks but to the stars are known,
But to the stars and the cold lunar beams;
Alone the sun arises, and alone
    Spring the great streams.

or more economically:

The cheerful silence of the fells.

The most notable examples of this natural imagery fused with the feeling it expresses are too long and too familiar for quotation—*Dover Beach* and *Isolation* (beginning "Yes, in the sea of life enisled"). Even more purely poetic is the expression of conflicting feelings not by pictures but by sound, in contrasting accents where we hear the altered tone:

Ye are bound for the mountains!
  Ah! with you let me go
Where your cold, distant barrier,
  The vast range of snow,
Through the loose clouds lifts dimly
  Its white peaks in air—
How deep is their stillness!
  Ah, would I were there!

But on the stairs what voice is this I hear
Buoyant as morning and as morning clear?
Say, has some wet bird-haunted English lawn
Lent it the music of its trees at dawn?
Or was it from some sun-fleck'd mountain brook
That the sweet voice its upland clearness took?

As magical and more majestic are the closing lines of *Sohrab and Rustum* and much of *Dover Beach.*

§3. By these illustrations I have tried to show how my own enjoyment of a poet depends upon his ability to communicate and my capacity to receive the expression of his moods and passion through language by the sensible images or more abstract ideas it invokes, and by the calming or exciting effect of metrical and accentual variations. The conclusion and the excuse of this long digression is to show that both the natural gift of vivid imagery and craftsmanship in poetical technique are useful, but only useful to the great purpose of communicating expressed emotion. The poet's real gift is "imaginative sympathy" in its two forms of insight into other minds and the projection of our feelings into nature or the recognition of their natural analogues therein. I am fortified in my confidence of interpreting Arnold's aim and genius correctly by his own description of a poet:

> Lean'd on his gate he gazes—tears
> Are in his eyes, and in his ears
> The murmur of a thousand years.
> Before him he sees life unroll,
> A placid and continuous whole—
> That general life, which does not cease,
> Whose secret is not joy but peace;
> That life, whose dumb aim is not miss'd
> If birth proceeds, if things subsist;
> The life of plants and stones and rain,
> The life he craves—if not in vain
> Fate gave, what chance shall not control,
> His sad lucidity of soul

or in a very different tone but with the same emotion recollected in tranquillity, still simple, sensuous, passionate:

> First hymn they the Father
> Of all things; and then
> The peace[1] of immortals,
> The action of men.
>
> The day in his hotness,
> The strife with the palm;
> The night in her silence,
> The stars in their calm.

[1]Arnold wrote "rest," but as that is ambiguous and I think commonly misunderstood with disastrous results, I have ventured correction. Cf. Ch. VI §9 note on Housman above.

§4. Swinburne I can treat much more briefly. He said more than Arnold though he had less to say. He had a greater flow of words and melody but less economy of management. Only in *Atalanta* and a few lyrics like *The Garden of Proserpine*, *Itylus*, *The Sea-mew* and *Ilicet* does he quite avoid tiring us; and the last title[1] might raise a smile in the profane at a lament so long drawn out, were its insistent repetitions not justified by the nature of the hopeless longing for "precious friends hid in death's dateless night" which they express. (*Quis desiderio sit pudor aut modus Tam cari capitis?*[2])

For all his fluency the themes of Swinburne's highest inspiration are comparatively few; chiefly the tragic transience of things, of youth and beauty, of love, of remembrance and of life; then freedom, not merely the political freedom of which he spoke so much, but the joy of untrammelled activity; and lastly one in which he has perhaps excelled all poets, the expression of maternal love. And similarly the sensible objects which he finds expressive of these passions are rather restricted in range; flowers, birds, the seasons and the sea are the most common. Shakespeare's Rosalind is perhaps an unsurpassed picture of graceful girlhood, but Swinburne's own confessed love of infants has helped him to his Althea, a portrait of motherhood unsurpassed by man or woman:

> For what lies light on many and they forget,
> Small things and transitory as a wind o' the sea,
> I forget never; I have seen thee all thine years
> A man in arms, strong and a joy to men
> Seeing thine head glitter and thine hand burn its way
> Through a heavy and iron furrow of sundering spears;
> But always also a flower of three suns old,
> The small one thing that lying drew down my life
> To lie with thee and feed thee; a child and weak,
> Mine, a delight to no man, sweet to me.

For the love of freedom the swimming episode from *Tristram of Lyonesse* may be cited and a few lines quoted from the *Sea-mew*.

[1]*Ire licet* = *Ite, missa est* (It is finished.)
[2]Who would blame or check our mourning for the loss of one so dear?

When I had wings, my brother,
Such wings were mine as thine

. . .

When loud with life that quakes,
The wave's wing spreads and flutters,
The wave's heart swells and breaks.

lines which also illustrate the two-way sympathy of imagination.

What emerges from a consideration of Swinburne is that his copious eloquence and marvellous fertility in new prosodic harmonies, when inspired by the tranquil contemplation of genuine passion, achieve an expressiveness in the first rank of poetry. When not so supported they sink into ornate garrulity or pathological crudeness.

§5. It has been well remarked that, in spite of their lovely episodes, the supreme beauties of the Homeric poems and of the Gospels, are the general effect of reading them as a whole. They express severally the half-nostalgic enthusiasm for the good old times, a "heroic age" already passed or passing, and the inspired longing for a kingdom that is yet to come. But in a degree this is true of many great poems which are also long. The gems of poetry which we linger over and quote lose half their brilliance when torn from the setting that has put us into the mood where "our affections gently lead us on."

Prose literature, like long poems, depends greatly on this power of producing an "atmosphere." Literal descriptions in terms of colour and shape are those which readers generally skip; good descriptions link the object to some feeling. "The cheerful silence of the fells," and Swinburne's description of the wave, both quoted above, really give us visions of nature, and the same method succeeds for human faces. Sounds can, of course, be described onomatopœically.

§6. Prose fiction, the widest of literary fields, must be treated more briefly. Much of what has been said about poetry, especially as narrative or dramatic, but also to some extent as lyrical, applies here. The necessity of sympathetic imagination, of entering into the beliefs and feelings of other people, is equally obvious, and the possession of this gift with the power of communicating the insight is alone almost the making of a novelist. Emphasis has often been laid upon "plot," "construction" and "action" as no less important than "character"; but to me at least, these are only means, perhaps the best means, of attaining the great end, the expression of feeling. Action is certainly a better revelation of character than an author's jejune psychological descriptions, or confessional harangues put into the mouths of the persons, but I doubt if it is more successful than such characteristic dialogue as that in which Jane Austen excels. Perhaps in all this I am peculiar, since I am unable to read the great majority of detective stories, all indeed which rely upon the solution of a problem without interesting me in the character of the parties. Whether X or Z, of whom I know little more than the difference of their finger-prints and foot-marks, committed the crime I cannot bring myself to care; I prefer a crossword puzzle. The *Sherlock Holmes* stories have always seemed to me the best in this kind, chiefly because they are unpretentiously short and because the author does invest his "problems" with an atmosphere of strange mystery and almost of "romance."

Tales of adventure I put in a higher class. At worst we can sympathize with the fears and triumphs of the hero and his hostility to the villain, but it is only when we get some deeper insight into the subtleties of character that we have works of art like Stevenson's *Kidnapped* and *Master of Ballantrae*[1] or Conrad's *Romance.* All these, together with tales of ancient times and foreign lands, of abnormal characters and mysterious experiences come under the heading of "strange" or "romantic,"[2] and I think the deepest distinction between works of fiction is between those which give us some understanding of the alien and those which give us one new and better of the familiar. In this latter kind Jane Austen is supreme, and I confess at once that I re-read her novels more often and with more delight than any others. Here are no characters or events strange to the average educated reader; everything depends upon the nicest discrimination of character and the

[1]*See Letters of H. James and R. L. Stevenson*, ed. J. A. Smith.
[2]*See* Appendix D.

subtlest expression of it in the characteristic language of the persons. Moreover the great dangers of a loose-girt form like the prose novel are exquisitely avoided—*longueurs*, didacticism, moralizing, the intrusion of the writer's personality or pose, everything that puts us out of key. Probably the greatest successor in this field is Henry James.[1] He fails of Jane Austen's beautiful lucidity, and in his attempt to illuminate the obscurer regions of the heart often only obscures them further; but he creates an atmosphere which is suitable to obscurity and he is almost as successful as she was in keeping himself out of sight. Katharine Mansfield shares this merit, and so does Virginia Woolf.[2]

In this last respect of self-exhibition gifted Victorian novelists from Thackeray to Meredith offended grievously. We should smile indulgently at Colonel Newcome and Amelia Sedley if Thackeray had not moralized till we are inclined to laugh. Meredith was perhaps unrivalled in expressing, as in *Harry Richmond* and *Beauchamp's Career*, the tragic tension between old and young who love one another and with both of whom we can sympathize; but his pretensions to "philosophy" and to wit are tedious and disgusting.

In the romantic or "strange" variety of fiction the humblest aspirant is the fairy-tale or tale of wonder, where there is impossible or improbable action. But how exquisite a success may be achieved when the *feelings* expressed are wholly natural is shown by Hans Andersen's *Wild Swans* and Rudyard Kipling's *Jungle Book*. More respected, though often less respectable, is the historical or foreign novel whose strangeness is merely that of time or space. Here there is apt to be a tawdry emphasis on externals and on shoddy archaisms, but, as usual, real imagination, like that of Sigred Undset's *Kristin Lavransdatter* and Rudyard Kipling's *Kim* and *Puck of Pook's Hill*, can make us at home in semi-barbarism. More ambitious still are the efforts at insight into the minds and hearts of a class inevitably alien to both the author and his readers, not because they are poorer, for they may be much richer, but because

[1]Partly by failure to conceal his artistry.

[2]Fielding's introductory Chapters are as good as the story, and little to do with it.

they are naturally inexpressive and uncommunicative: children, illiterates, or slaves to wealth or poverty. Such are the best novels of Wells, Arnold Bennett and Steinbeck. In many of these attempts the difficulty is overcome by the elaboration of background. The persons are explained to us by their setting in a social or political atmosphere which prepares us for their peculiarity. Exactly opposite is the method of the highest ideal of strangeness, the strangeness of a rare individuality, saint or criminal or genius, near allied to madness, like Dostoievski's Alyosha and Raskolnikoff. Here our imagination is conciliated by shutting all windows on the out-door world and closeting us with the abnormal so closely that we come to accept it. Each method has its dangers, its failures and its triumphs. Flaubert's *Madame Bovary* is a curiously isolated presentment of an obsession so commonplace that in its isolation from the common life it becomes, to me, fantastic. Duhamel in his *Chronique des Pasquier*, I think, succeeds in both methods; his unimaginative characters are illuminated by their social setting, his rarer minds are set apart in a rarer atmosphere; all live in a great world.

The purpose of this brief and personal review has been to substantiate my contention that almost the whole of my great pleasure in novel-reading comes from the imaginative sympathy it gives me with the minds of others, and the consequent insight into my own.

CHAPTER XIV

CLASSICAL AND ROMANTIC CRITICISM

§1. The method originally laid down for our procedure was to test our hypothesis as to the nature of æsthetic experience empirically. An attempt has been made to do this first by drawing on the most trustworthy report of experience, that of introspection. It remains to check this by the reports of other persons, restricting ourselves of necessity to some selected field. The inevitable restriction may be made with regard to both time and subject. The time should preferably be not our own day, where it is hard to avoid the bias of fashion in assessing the importance of the material.

§2. Probably no period was so rich in attempts to make intelligible to itself the nature of its æsthetic experience as the eighteenth century, especially in our own country. The Greek writers had much curiosity but inadequate variety of experience upon which to employ it. With the art of Christianity, of the Middle Ages and of the Renaissance the diversity of matter became immensely stimulating, but only after the Cartesian renewal of philosophy did the growth of æsthetic theory begin to accelerate. Then within about a century we get a surprisingly rich harvest: Addison, Hutcheson, Burke, Hume, Hogarth, Alison, Reynolds, Home, Kant, Coleridge, Wordsworth, all threw some new light on the problem which had already been raised by Socrates or Plato, though their treatment of it had hardly been advanced in the long interval. The reason for this sudden revival, and also for its peculiar relevance to our inquiry, is that the eighteenth-century writers invented, or first clearly recognized, a contrast and even a hostility between two tendencies or, as they were tempted to say, two kinds of art, a controversy which is most instructive as to the nature of æsthetic experience in general. The growth of this consciousness was doubtless due to the revolution and counter-revolution in taste and artistic creation between, say, the Elizabethans and Pope and between Pope and Shelley.

§3. The predominance of the words "classical" and "romantic" in modern criticism with any pretensions to a theoretical basis must surely indicate something of importance for æsthetics, however loose and worthless the ways in which they are commonly used. The thought which lies behind them perhaps first found a stimulus in the contrast between the orthodox tradition of Aristotle's *Poetics*, or Vitruvius, and the exciting rediscovery of the treatise on *Sublimity* ascribed to Longinus. This contrast, as it was generally exaggerated, may be roughly summarized as one between the emphasis on form of composition and that on the loftiness or passion or strangeness of the theme. The comparison of these two classical authorities formulated itself in one of the dreariest of artistic controversies, that between the adherents of the Ancients and the Moderns, a controversy which even Swift's[1] cavalier treatment could hardly rescue from dullness.

In less pedantic or more historical critics the terms of controversy soon changed to "Gothic," with the connotation of "rude" or barbarous, and "classical" connoting regularity. It was not long before the disputants contended under the more equal standards of "classical" and "romantic."

§4. The attempt to make clearer the real and important distinction underlying our vague usage of these terms to-day, and so to use them more precisely, may best be furthered by some consideration of their history.[2] "Classical" is of course the older term. In Latin it meant a citizen fully enfranchised on a property qualification as distinct from one whose only stake in the State was his children. Gellius, however, applies it to literature: *Auctor classicus et assiduus, non proletarius.*[3]

The Oxford English Dictionary gives us the earliest relevant application—that of Sandys who in 1599 speaks of "classicall and canonical" writings. In 1613 we hear of those which are "classic, chief and approved," but subsequently the implication

[1]*The Battle of the Books*. Cf. H. Rigault, *La querelle des anciens et des modernes* (Paris, 1856).

[2]*See* Appendix D for historical instances.

[3]One who writes like a scholar and a gentleman, not like a boor.

is of similarity either in style or substances to the Greek and Roman authors. So Collins in 1744 says:

And classic judgment gain'd to sweet Racine
The temperate strength of Maro's chaster line.

Johnson gives two meanings (1) "relating to antique authors" and (2) "of the first order or rank." "Romantic" likewise at first meant similar for style or subject to the romances or novels popular in the seventeenth century.

§5. From this derivation and from the earlier quotations given in Appendix D it seems that the first idea associated with the word romantic was what Pater calls the addition of strangeness to beauty, a strangeness which might for Pepys be mere "incredibility." As Fénelon says in 1714 "Pour les héros des romans ils n'ont rien de naturel; ils sont faux, doucereux et fades." And falseness or affectation has always been the besetting sin of romance as Saint Beuve diagnosed it "L'écueil particulier du genre romantique c'est le faux." Sometimes the strangeness was merely that of distance in time or place:

'Tis distance lends enchantment to the view
And robes the mountain in its azure hue.[1]

§6. Only gradually was the idea added that this strangeness, again in Pater's words, must be "drawn from the deep places of the imagination." For, after all, neither the merely strange, such as a week's continuous rain or a five-legged sheep, nor the merely old or distant, such as coal from Australia, need have any æsthetic value. Classical architecture is older than Gothic—which was almost synonymous with both barbarous and romantic—but as Reynolds[2] acutely remarked, speaking of his own times and circle, "Gothic architecture though not so ancient as the Grecian, is more so to our imagination, with which the artist is more concerned than with absolute truth." If the æsthetic meaning of imagination is not merely

[1]Campbell, *Pleasures of Hope*.
[2]*Royal Academy Lecture XIII* (1786).

the power of vivid visualization but the sympathetic realization of other people's feelings,[1] it is easy to see how the attempt to express and communicate the alien feelings of different ages, races, sex and classes has its difficulties and dangers, but also its striking triumphs which were neither desired nor deserved by an "age of reason." What is strange is *exciting*, what is familiar is *restful*, what is beautiful is the expression of *emotion* recollected in *tranquillity*; these are the two elements present in all æsthetic experience, perfectly balanced in its perfection but more often in some disequilibrium.

§7. Croce[2] shows very well the relevance of all this to his own formula for æsthetic experience, which, as has been said, is very similar to my own:

"The answer (to our problem) may be said to emerge as the result of criticizing the greatest contest of conflicting tendencies ever waged in the field of art, a conflict waged not only in the age when it was most conspicuous and to which it gave its name: the conflict of classicism and romanticism. Romanticism demands from art above all things a spontaneous torrent of emotion, love and hatred, anguish and triumph, despair and rapture. It is contented, even delighted, with vague and misty images, a suggestive and unequal style, dim hints, approximations of phrase, violent, turbid outlines. Classicism, on the other hand, loves the serene soul, the learned design, figures studied in their character and precise in line; deliberation, balance, lucidity. It sets its face resolutely towards truth as romanticism did towards feeling. And a host of reasons can be found for maintaining either point of view. For what, ask the romantics, is an art worth, for all its polished imagery, that does not speak to our hearts? And if it speak to our hearts what matter if its imagery is unpolished? And their enemies will answer them: What is this emotional excitement worth when the mind can find no lovely imagery to rest in? And if the imagery be lovely, what matters the lack of a passion attainable without the help of art, showered upon us by life often more freely than we could wish? . . .

[1]*See* Chapter IX.

[2]*Breviario di Estetica*, translated by D. Ainslie, *Essentials of Æsthetic*. The rendering is my own.

Great artists and great work, or at least the great parts of it, can be called neither classicist nor romantic; for they are both classical and romantic, emotional and life-like, they are sheer emotion absolutely identified with the most lucid imagery."

§8. All this is well borne out in the use made of metre by so-called classical and romantic poets severally, and by their theories of its uses. On the one hand we have highly regular rhythms, either blank verse or, more characteristically, the heroic couplet as in Pope. On the other we have either completely irregular "verse" or the most exquisite research for diversity and divergence which shall suit and enhance the passion, as often in Shelley. On the one hand Dryden[1] says: "The excellence and dignity of rime . . . which I consider most in it, because I have not seldom found it, is that it bounds and circumscribes the fancy. For imagination in a poet is a faculty so wild and lawless, that like a high-ranging spaniel, it must have clogs tied to it, lest it outrun the judgment. The great easiness of blank verse renders the poet too luxuriant." On the other hand Wordsworth[2] says: "Metre will be found greatly to contribute to impart passion to the words." And more impartially Coleridge:[3] "Passion itself imitates order, and the order resulting produces a pleasurable passion, and thus (poetry) elevates the mind by making its feelings the object of its reflexion. So likewise, whilst it recalls the sights and sounds that had accompanied the occasions of the original passions, it . . . yet tempers the passion by the calming power which all distinct images exert in the human soul."

The romantic element in all *æsthetic experience* is the passion, the classical or tranquil element is its contemplation and expression. In the *work of art* the technique of communication must be included.

[1]Preface to *The Rival Ladies* (1664, the first play in heroic couplets or sixty years).

[2]Preface to *Lyrical Ballads* (1800).

[3]*On Poesy or Art* (1818).

CHAPTER XV

FORM AND SUBJECT IN POETRY[1]

A Question Prior to an Æsthetic of Poetry

§1. The solution of the problem now to be discussed would affect some of the preceding arguments and conclusions. But since it could not profitably be discussed till the meaning of its terms had been analysed, and since moreover I am very doubtful of the solution, I have postponed the discussion to this place.

Roger Fry in *Last Lectures* threw out the suggestion that the inferiority of neolithic to palæolithic painting might be due to the birth or growth of language and the consequent temptation to dull the vivid sensibility for individual experiences by the practically useful habit of abstract or generalized thinking. Whether or no the birth and growth of language involved a set-back for graphic and plastic art, it certainly first made poetry possible. And the question which puzzles me is this: Would any art analogous to poetry have been possible without speech? What if a tongue-tied race had invented a system of ideograms or purely conventional gestures?

I suppose the first stage would have been that anybody wanting a knife might have drawn a schematic knife in the sand and made a gesture of grasping. Then, if in some obviously unpractical situation, say in the absence of enemies or of the other sex, they had gone through the gestures of courtship or of battle, we should have the love- or war-dance, the pure mime, supposed to be the forerunner of lyric and of drama. If they had next drawn a set of such gestures, we should have had the germ of anecdotal, historical, illustrative, "heroic" painting, that *genre* which Reynolds thought the noblest of his art, that "poetic" element which some modern theorists

[1]This chapter has been reproduced, with some alteration, by the Editor's leave, from *Philosophy*, January, 1941.

would banish from painting to the silent film. That both the acted and the painted mime would have been arts seems clear, but even clearer that neither would have been poetry, which must include real or imagined vocal sounds. Indeed, rigorous iconoclasts are found to demand that even from poetry all its significance or reference, all elements except the purely formal one of sound, should be eliminated.

§2. Suppose, then, a further step. Suppose that instead of more or less realistic pictures of persons acting or of natural objects, these speechless artists had invented a system of pure ideograms, in which persons, things, qualities, actions, events, relations, were symbolized by visual signs with no more intrinsic relation to the thing signified than musical notation has to the tune, or my car-number to my character, but also with no suggestion of any spoken words. This, I suppose, would be what writing is to a man born stone-deaf. Could such a system of reference be used for artistic purposes? Could it achieve beauty? I am tempted to think it could, though certainly not poetry. It is hard for us to imagine such a usage, for we have all talked before we could read, so that writing seems essentially to presuppose speech. But we are told that there has actually existed in China an ideography which could be quite indifferently read off into several spoken languages and having no special affinity to any one. Certainly in 1668 Bishop Wilkins, in his *Essay Towards a Real Character and a Philosophical Language*, proposed "the expression of our conceptions by Marks which shall signify things not Words." Leibniz in his *De Re Combinatoria* seems to have had the same idea.

To a small extent what happened in China happens in our own experience. "X" can equally be read as ten or *zehn* or *dix* (and conversely all these can equally be symbolized by 10). "&" is no more "and" than it is "et" or "und" or "e." The best modern instances of ideogram are no doubt the signs of number, mensuration, and mathematical operation: (÷ + √); but fairly complicated ideas not closely connected with any linguistic signs are represented by dashes, parentheses ("this is by the way"), inverted commas ("these are the words he used"), notes of interrogation ("this is a question"), and the use of capitals (either "this is a new thought" or "this is a proper name").[1]

§3. If, then, we ask whether such pure ideography could be used with artistic effect, on the one hand we feel inclined to answer, Yes; for by its means surely there might be brought before the minds of the deaf and dumb the very same human experiences and aspirations which are brought to us by poetry, whether in prose or verse, or by a mime. On the other hand, we feel driven to say, No; for in all those arts the sensuous quality of some medium, either sound or gesture, whether actual or imagined, seems necessary to the æsthetic effect; but here we must assume that the sensible nature of the ideograms would be as irrelevant as the fount of type used in printing Shakespeare or the colour of the ink in which Mozart is scored. Either of these might give a slight æsthetic pleasure, but this would not fuse with the music or the poetry, as sounds do with sense; it would be just as beautiful if it recorded doggerel.

On the other hand, the sound of a verse, though it often seems to contribute as much as anything to its beauty, may be trivial if we are quite ignorant of the meaning, or if that meaning, by a negligible change of sound, is much altered. Consider the classical controversy over the phrase:

> Our noisy years seem moments in the being
> Of the eternal silence.

Saintsbury (*History of English Prosody*, iii. 74–7) maintained that the beauty of the sound was quite independent of the meaning. But he spoiled his case by a malicious paraphrase,

[1]It is obvious that the same written signs may suggest either different sounds and ideas to different nations ("pain"), or the same sound and different ideas to one nation ("ball"). The same written signs are very differently pronounced by a Cockney and a Tynesider: (Doctor: "Can you walk yet?" Patient: "Work! I can't even walk!"). I pronounce Greek rather differently from some of my friends, and so, I presume, did an Athenian from a Syracusan. Conversely, "cougher" and "coffer" represent to an Englishman the same sounds but different ideas. "BAG" and "bag" the same sound and the same idea.

intended to show that with an identical meaning the beauty might vanish:

> Our $\left\{\begin{matrix}\text{loud-sounding}\\ \text{clamorous}\end{matrix}\right\}$ twelvemonths appear $\left\{\begin{matrix}\text{minutes}\\ \text{seconds}\end{matrix}\right\}$ in
> The unending soundlessness.

It is a pity he could not resist this. The substitution of precise terms for more colloquial generalized words with vaguer connotations either changes or destroys the meaning. "Noisy music" does not mean the same as "loud-sounding music." Everybody would know what "our noisy years" meant, but I should attach no meaning at all to "our clamorous twelve months." And it seems impossible to conceive how a loud-sounding twelve months could appear to be a second in a soundlessness of any duration.

So against this Andrew Bradley's contention (*Poetry for Poetry's Sake*) is undeniable, that the beauty of the sound depends almost entirely on some subtle adjustment to the meaning. But Bradley goes further. Perhaps in reaction against Saintsbury's unfairness, he seems to allow that the meaning of the paraphrase *is* the same and to conclude that, since that has no beauty, the beauty lies wholly in the union of the two, and the mere meaning has as little as the mere sound. That mere meaning has no strictly *poetic* beauty must be granted, but has it none? Take a fairer paraphrase, such as might be offered by an intelligent schoolboy: "All the turmoil of our lives is a brief episode in the endless tenor of the universe." Or substitute a different poem:

> We are such stuff
> As dreams are made on, and our little lives
> Are rounded with a sleep.

or

> πάντα γέλως καὶ πάντα κόνις καὶ πάντα τὸ μηδέν.[1]

§4. Have not all these something in common which has æsthetic value, something which I can only describe as the

[1]*See* Appendix C., p. 140 for translation.

contemplation of the human tragedy, something which would also be indicated without metaphor or simile in the vernacular "It will be all the same a thousand years hence" or "We must all die"?[1] It will probably be replied that all these phrases have different meanings, that they have nothing æsthetically in common. We must therefore take instances of deliberate translation and choose instances where the translators, believing that they were dealing with inspired meanings, have striven to present the same meaning. I will take two such sets of instances, where, in my view, there is an element of meaning common to the instances already quoted:

(1) A thousand years in thy sight are but as yesterday, seeing that is past as a watch in the night (Ps. xc. 4, Prayer Book Version).

χίλια ἔτη ἐν ὀφθαλμοῖς σου ὡς ἡ ἡμέρα ἡ ἐχθὲς ἥτις διῆλθε, καὶ φυλακὴ ἐν νυκτί.

Nam mille annos si praetereat, sunt in oculis tuis ut dies hesternus vigiliaque nocturna.

(2) As for man, his days are as grass; as a flower of a field, so he flourisheth (Ps. ciii. 15).

ἄνθρωπος ὡσεὶ χόρτος αἱ ἡμέραι αὐτοῦ, ὡσεὶ ἄνθος τοῦ ἀγροῦ οὕτως ἐξανθήσει.

Ipsius mortalis similes faeno dies esse, sic ut flos agri, sic florere ipsum.

In set (1) and again in set (2) the sounds are quite different in the different tongues, but I think it clear that in each set there is an identical core of meaning which has a recognizable æsthetic quality. I should myself say that the two sets also share such an identical core, which is also identical with that of the passages quoted earlier; that in all there is also an identical æsthetic quality which is different from the æsthetic quality common to such a pair of passages as:

[1]There is great poetic significance, to which the sound of the words contributes little, especially when they are not spoken by an Irish actor, in the conclusion of Synge's *Riders to the Sea:* "No man at all can live for ever and we must be satisfied."

Bliss was it in that dawn to be alive,
But to be young was very heaven.

and

The delightful commerce of the world
. . . .
When we were young, when we could number friends
In all the Italian cities like ourselves.

§5. Now if the ideographic technique I have imagined should exist, which could indicate or refer to things and our experiences of them directly, without the intermediate reference to vocal sounds, and if this technique were employed by an artist obsessed by the same sort of experience which was obsessing the writers of all those passages about death, would he produce a beautiful work of art? And if so, would it be just a different work, differing from theirs as they differ from one another and as a carved crucifix differs from a painting, or would it be of a totally novel kind, in that it would make directly the reference that they make indirectly, sharing indeed their common reference, but dispensing with any sensuous æsthetic medium such as they all have? Would it be only like looking at an object through a different coloured glass, or rather like touching it for the first time? And if the latter, would this substitution of (as it were) tangibility for visibility mean a total loss of beauty, or the substitution of a different beauty, or the apprehension face to face of a beauty we had previously seen through various glasses darkly?

When Kant said that the moral law within him was sublime, he clearly ascribed to it or to its contemplation an æsthetic character. And he surely did not think that this in any degree depended upon the sound of the words *Moralisches Gesetz*. No doubt his æsthetics distinguished sublimity from beauty as not depending for its æsthetic value upon form. And we might feel tempted to say that the æsthetic experience communicated by the ideographic artist would be sublime. But if the contemplation of death or martyrdom is sublime, might not that of youth or happy love be beautiful? Might not the contemplation of some passionate or dramatic episode in my own youth or among my neighbours or in historical or imaginary persons have æsthetic quality? And might not my attention be directed and focused upon it by symbols totally lacking in æsthetic quality or at least with none that could fuse with that of the experience indicated?[1] And if so, would not the use of these symbols be an art? And if so, would it be just another art, or would it, for better or worse, be unique? Does a man born deaf have an æsthetic experience in reading poetry, and, if so, is it like any we have?[2]

§6. Helen Keller, blind and stone-deaf from infancy, said she enjoyed poetry much more after she had acquired speech (i.e., I suppose, had learnt to associate certain motor sensations of the larynx with tactile symbols). A verse of her own composition is given:

The forest trees have donned
Their gorgeous autumn tapestries,
  A mysterious hand is silently stripping the trees.
And with rustle and whirr the leaves descend
And, like little frightened birds,
  Lie trembling on the ground.

She said that she knew that "rustle" and "whirr" were onomatopœic and explained the meaning of that word, but I suppose she only knew this in the way in which she knew that autumn tapestries were gorgeous. When asked whether she thought more in finger language or in vocal language, she replied: "I think my thoughts as I spell them on my fingers." Whether either of these motor sensations would be more capable of

[1]Had a medieval knight contemplating an escutcheon any æsthetic experience, comparable perhaps to that of reading the *Forsyte Saga*? Cf. Lamb's feelings in face of the escutcheon at Blakesmoor (*Last Essays of Elia* i.)

[2]Consider an analogy. A blind man or a man with his eyes shut certainly apprehends no beauty in a rainbow, and surely not the same in a rose or a statuette that we do. Is the beauty which it is claimed he can feel in a statuette like what we see there or more like what we might feel in a delightful fabric or a delightful breeze, or, again, more like what we might feel in reading:

"Perfect little body without fault or stain on thee,
  With promise of strength and manhood full and fair,"

or *Vera incessu patuit dea?* (Her step revealed a true divinity.)

fusing with the experiences they referred to than a written ideography I cannot tell.[1]

No doubt an ideogram would acquire by association the suggestion of emotions usually accompanying the thing it signified, and this might come to seem natural, especially to the deaf and dumb who had no verbal communication, and who would indeed think in ideograms. But, on our assumption that the ideograms were in no degree pictorial, it is hard to see how any calligraphic beauty they or their arrangement might possess could fuse with the beauty of the meaning as vocal sounds often can, though the meaning of these too was originally in part conventional. The human voice is in itself more meaningful than pen strokes.

§7. In answer to the question whether an ideographic symbolism could achieve beauty, all my æsthetic presuppositions incline me to answer, No, just because it would be quite arbitrary and conventional. The medium or "form" would be indifferent; as we have seen that musical notation might be altered and nothing of the music changed, whereas in poetry translation gives a different poem or none.[2] And I have always believed that beauty consisted in the fusion of a sensuous image with an inner experience which it expressed, so that the expression seemed as inevitable as a smile. But here there would be no such fusion. This belief of mine was shared by Bradley, and a few more sentences from the same essay will elaborate it better than I can. He is protesting against the antithesis of a sheer subject-matter and a sheer form as rivals for the ownership of the beauty of a poem. He suggests that such a subject-matter would be "something real or imaginary, for instance the Fall of Man, as it exists in the minds of fairly cultivated people," and this subject, he points out, is not to be found in *Paradise Lost*, and therefore cannot be that in which the beauty of the poem consists. He accordingly sub-

[1]American Association to Promote the Teaching of Speech to Deaf Mutes, Report of Fourth Summer Meeting, Chatauqua, N.Y., 1894. "H. Keller," by J. McFarland.

[2]Cf. "Les traductions sont comme les femmes; quand elles sont belles elles ne sont pas fidèles, et quand elles sont fidèles elles ne sont pas belles."

stitutes an antithesis between two elements which *are* to be found in the poem, one which he calls the substance, for instance the events, characters, and scenes in *Paradise Lost*, and the other the form or measured language in which they are described. And he maintains that to ask in which of these the beauty of the poem lies is absurd, because neither without the other could be what it is. "They are one thing from different points of view and in that sense identical." "The experience is of something in which the two are absolutely fused." I will not for the present contest that this is true of any *poetic* experience. Let it be granted that the expressions τετέλεσται, "it is finished," "consummatum est" (St. John xix. 30) and κεκαρτέρηται τἄμα (*Eur. Hipp.* 1455) just have different beauties and that it is vain to ask whether their beauties depend more upon the similar experiences they express or upon the different sounds which express them. I am still driven to question the corollary, implied by Bradley and more explicit in Croce and others, that *all* æsthetic experience essentially involves such an indissoluble fusion of substance or fact referred to and sensuous form or means of reference. Could there not be a way of suggesting or stimulating an æsthetic activity in which the referring medium was quite indifferent and in which the value therefore depended wholly on the experience stimulated or referred to? Here, I think, Bradley himself falters. He admits that, if I have forgotten every single word of *Hamlet*, I may retain something, though not all, of the actions and characters which are the substance of the poem and, in a sense, in it. Nor, he says, does he question the poetic value, in a wide sense of "poetic" (he means æsthetic), of all this even when thought of apart from the poem. He compares it to "our recollections of the heroes of history or legend, who move about in our imagination, and are worth much to us, though we do not remember anything they said." Professor Gilbert Murray has somewhere pointed out that the reading of the Gospels, whether in Greek or English, or of Homer, even in a good translation, leaves in our minds something of æsthetic value, a picture of "the Homeric world" or of "the Kingdom," though we cannot quote a passage. As Bradley again puts it: "We may forget all the words and not profess to remember even the 'meaning,' but believe that we possess the 'spirit' of the poem. And what we possess may have an immense value, though the poem, of course, it is not." And again: "We may find analogues to the meaning of a poem outside it. The other arts, the best ideas of philosophy or religion, much that nature and life offer us or force upon us, are akin to it, though only akin."

§8. In spite, then, of a deep-seated philosophic reluctance, I have been driven to ask whether after all there may not be something in a Hegelian distinction which, in the past, under the influence of Croce and to some extent of Bradley himself, I have been apt to ridicule.[1] Hegel holds[2] that in a poem there are three distinguishable elements, each having æsthetic quality:

(i) The subject-matter or content (*Inhalt*, *Sache*), which must itself be poetical. This, I think, is Bradley's rejected "subject."

(ii) The "idea" or presentation (*Vorstellung*), equivalent, I suppose to Bradley's "substance," which must be a poetical "idea."

(iii) The verbal expression of this, which must be a poetical expression.

For instance, he says that the words

Als nun die dämmernde Eos mit Rosenfingern emporstieg

and the words

Ἦμος δ' ἠριγένεια φάνη ῥοδοδάκτυλος Ἠώς.

are different poetical expressions of the *same* poetical presentation; which is itself only one poetical presentation of a poetic content of which, I suppose,

The morn in russet mantle clad

would express another presentation.

[1] *Theory of Beauty*, VII, §§ 11, 12.
[2] *Æsthetik*, III, pp. 227, 244–5, 270–7.

I hesitate to accept this analysis as it stands. But it does seem as if we must make our account with at least two æsthetic elements fused in a poem but each capable of æsthetic existence outside that fusion:

(i) An æsthetic "substance" not yet vocalized or visualized. The beauty of this may be slight.

(ii) The sensible or imagined sounds by which such an idea may be indicated, referred to, or expressed. These sounds may have some beauty of their own.

In a poem these two separate beauties would be fused and produce one probably much greater than the sum of the two.

If we wished to justify Hegel's triple analysis, which makes the imagination of certain bare facts "poetical" (or rather æsthetic) as distinguished from that of others which is not, I suppose we might say that human emotions are the poetic facts. Perhaps they alone and always are things capable of æsthetic contemplation. It is not the relative positions of a star and a planet, but an experience, promise, foreboding, or parting—which is dawn.

Of these three elements, ideography clearly could give us the first. It could focus our attention on the fact that men lose what they love or that Orpheus lost Eurydice. Would that in itself be beautiful? It could also give us the second—metaphor, simile, and such "figures." Would that be sufficient, or would it be necessary, for beauty? Part of the third it clearly could not give us—rhyme, rhythm, metre, assonance, alliteration, onomatopœia. That it could give us part of the third (antithesis, repetition, parallelism, and several figures for which Greek rhetoricians invented queer names) is a fact I have neglected as obscuring the issue I want to raise: Can there be art without form?

CHAPTER XVI

CONCLUSION

THE argument here set out may be summarized as follows: Beauty, though we unreflectively ascribe it to things and sensa, cannot really be one of their qualities. We ascribe it to those which have a certain significance or expression *for us*. But significance or expression is a relation between that which expresses and the mind to which it expresses or which expresses itself in it. There may be a third term in the relation, when one mind expresses or communicates its experiences to another by physical media. But what a natural object or artifact signifies to me must depend on my character and history at least as much as on its own. The reality we are dealing with when we talk of beauty is æsthetic experience. But not all claims to æsthetic experience are justified; they may have degrees of vivacity and purity or may have quite falsely assumed the name. Some people call beautiful what they think true or edifying or useful or sensuously agreeable, and nothing else. This is to have bad taste. Some hardly recognize any beauty. This is to have little taste. The æsthetic experience is to find some perception or sensuous image significant of emotion, not an arbitrary symbol of it, not a mere symptom, nor an inducement of it, but an expression of it, as words can be expressive of thoughts or a smile of affection. And the æsthetic expericnce is not the expression of thought nor the communication of such expression, nor that of sensation, nor yet that of acts of choice. It is the expression of an emotion in an individual mind; and the communication of this expression to other minds is the work of art, and this needs technique.

All this seems obviously true of poetry but less obvious of natural beauty and of other arts, especially those which are unrepresentative. Yet if we are right in calling all these experiences by one name—"beautiful" or "æsthetic"—and if expression is the essential character of one, it must be of all. And both the authority of the best critics and examination of my own experience reassures me that so it is. To the question how it is that sensuous things are naturally expressive of emotion answers have been essayed by metaphysics and perhaps more plausibly by various sciences—physiology, psychology, anthropology, sociology—and, for the individual, by biographical history.

In support of the contention that all æsthetic experiences, where we use the expression "beautiful" in its ordinary sense, really have a common character or relation (that of expressing emotion) we may adduce the failure of all attempts to distinguish accurately "kinds" of beauty. Of these the most plausible is that of "representative" and "formal" beauty, of which the first is supposed to remind us by resemblance or association of pleasant objects and the other to please merely by its sensuous surface. Yet both are called "significant," both are closely connected with emotion, and it seems true that the connection is one of expression. Natural beauties sometimes elude this distinction. Another popular classification is that of classical and romantic beauty (or beauty and sublimity), but any attempt to divide æsthetic experiences on those lines ends in confusion. The underlying truth of this, as of the previously mentioned attempt, seems to be that in any expression of emotion both emotion and expression are concerned and may be unevenly balanced. When the emotion is not mastered we have the romantic, which may be false and crude; when it is deficient we have the classical, which may be cold.

The genius required for great works of art is commonly called imagination. And some degree of this faculty, which can hardly be quite absent in any man, is admittedly required for the appreciation of both art and nature. But the term is vague. Mere vividness of memory, visual, auditory or other, and even readiness in combining such mental images, may be very useful but are not all that is required for æsthetic experience, any more than keen eyesight or a good ear, probably more common in animals than in ourselves. The power to recover our past emotions—love, sorrow, indignation, hope, seems more important. We could never express nor comprehend the expression of emotions of which we had no experience whatever. For a purely lyric artist perhaps this power of realizing the nature of emotions to which he is not at the moment a prey might seem enough. But it has commonly been held that he can only express them, even to himself, in some sensuous form—in imagined shapes, colours, sounds and perhaps scents and tastes—and can only communicate his experience to others in physical instances of these. Some reasons for doubting this have been suggested in the last chapter.

At any rate it is clear that even the lyric artist commonly uses for the expression of his emotions the suggestion of natural objects whether by simile and metaphor or by direct allusion, and most often imputes to these objects some kind of feelings in sympathy with his own—happiness to the lark, sadness to the moon, anger to the waves, youth to the bud. Certainly the success of the dramatic artist depends upon imaginative sympathy with the emotions of his fellow-men, "putting himself in the place of others and of many others." The æsthetic experience seems to be not the criticism of life, nor its theory nor its furtherance—terms proper to morals, to science and to mental or physical hygiene—but the sympathetic contemplation of its delights and of its tragedy. *Humani nil a se alienum putat.*

APPENDIX A

TRANSCENDENTAL FEELING

THE idea that in æsthetic experience we attain a greater amount of truth than by thinking, or truth about more important matters, has been so often and so vaguely expressed that perhaps the best way of clearing our minds on the subject is to examine in detail one of the few modern attempts to give it a precise formulation.

Professor Stewart explains the "transcendental feeling" which he claims is excited by all great art or natural beauty as "a solemn sense of the overshadowing presence of 'That which was, and is, and ever shall be'."[1] He also describes it as "dream consciousness" and as "timeless." It is produced by "the persistence in us of that primeval condition from which we are sprung, when Life was still as sound asleep as death, and there was no Time yet." The principle of this life is "the Vegetative Part of the Soul" which "silently makes the assumption that Life is worth living." It is a "solemn sense of Timeless Being." "Such feeling . . . is rightly called Transcendental, because it is not one of the effects, but the condition of our entering upon that course of endeavour which makes experience."[2]

In this exposition of his subject the author throws together a number of characters which, so far from being connected, appear even mutually inconsistent.

(1) In what sense is the experience "timeless"? It presumably occurs at a date and lasts for a period which begins and ends. Nor does it seem to be an experience of something timeless for it is said to be of what "was and is and ever shall be." It does not seem to be e.g., an experience of logical

[1]*The Myths of Plato*, p. 36 and following.

[2]A subtler, or at least more elusive form of the theory seems adumbrated in Mr. Day Lewis's *The Poetic Image*, which contains many sensitive and penetrating remarks by the way.

connections which might be called timeless. What can be meant by a *primeval* condition *before* there was Time?

(2) Why is it called a "dream consciousness"? My own dreams are almost invariably very prosaic affairs, about events in time and much like real life, but less connected. I have on one occasion, under anæsthetic, believed that I was contemplating some kind of orrery and its contemplation filled me with an intense conviction of understanding something of immense importance[1] or perhaps everything. This experience was delusively logical rather than æsthetic; it is not common in dreams, not timeless, and something like it can occur when we are in our right mind.

(3) Why should it be said that such experiences belong to "the Vegetative part of the soul," that is to say that they are common to cabbages and perhaps toad-stools, from whom we may be descended? What is meant by the suggestion that vegetables "silently assume that life is worth living"? Is it merely meant that they do live? But they also die.

Some of the loose language which is here paradoxically used to describe all æsthetic experiences might, I think, be, with equal looseness but more plausibly, applied to some of them, though I doubt if all of it could be applied to any one. Some æsthetic experiences are rather like some dreams, indeed some are dreams; some obscure our sense of time's passage, as do some unæsthetic experiences, and some seem to refer to undated events; all may be called non-logical in the sense that they do not profess to be historically, scientifically or morally true, but this is so with many unæsthetic experiences which yet are not vegetative; some suggest the joy of life but others the blackness of despair.

Some of the poetic passages which Professor Stewart quotes in support of this thesis do seem to me to be loosely describable by some of these epithets, none by all, and some by none. I could add to the last class:

> And yet what days were those Parmenides!
> When we were young, when we could number friends
> In all the Italian cities like ourselves.[2]

[1]Addington Symonds related a similar experience.
[2]M. Arnold, *Empedocles.*

or

Life's . . . a tale
Told by an idiot, full of sound and fury,
Signifying nothing.[1]

or

As fair art thou, my bonnie lass,
So deep in luve am I:
And I will luve thee still, my dear,
Till a' the seas gang dry.[2]

No doubt the feelings arising from such convictions as Stewart here indicates may be strong and may be æsthetically expressed, as may Burns's conviction that he would be constant. But neither conviction nor expression is any evidence of philosophical or prophetic truth; constancy is not timeless nor remarkable in vegetables; philosophy is remarkable neither in vegetables nor in dreams. Any emotion seems capable of æsthetic expression.

APPENDIX B

BEAUTY AS THE EXPRESSION OF EMOTION

To show how naturally this has been felt in all ages to be the nature of beauty it may be of interest to collect some striking passages. The quotations are not literal but abbreviated.[3]

Plato, *Republic*, 400D–402.—Good style and harmony and grace and rhythm spring naturally from goodness of nature. The art of

[1]Shakespeare, *Macbeth* V. v.
[2]Burns.
[3]*See* my *Philosophies of Beauty from Socrates to Robert Bridges*, index. Pope says, "The proper study of mankind is man"; Wordsworth speaks of "The mind of man, the haunt and the main region of my song."

design is full of such qualities, in the fashioning of embroidery and architecture and not least of human bodies. 500—Harmony in music is expressive of character.

Timæus, 47—We might apply the geometrical motions of the heavenly bodies to the motions of our own minds which are akin to them. The movements of melody and rhythm are related to the changes of our own souls.

Aristotle, *Problems*, xix. 38.—We delight in melody because it expresses dispositions, and rhythm because it moves us in a regular way..

Politics, V (viii) 5.—When we hear "imitations" we all experience sympathetic feelings.

"Longinus" *On the Sublime*, viii—Nothing is so eloquent as real passion. ix. Sublimity is the echo of a great soul. xxxix. The flute can communicate passion to its hearers and compel them to identify themselves with the melody.

Plotinus, *Enneads*, V. viii. 2.—In beauty we see the reflection of our own spirits.

J. Dennis, *The Advancement of Modern Poetry*.I.—There must be passion everywhere in poetry and painting 'Tis the expression of this passion which gives us so much pleasure in authors.

Muratori, *The Perfection of Poetry*, xv.—We imagine or create images when excited by passion, and mostly picture lifeless things as alive.

Lord Shaftesbury, *Characteristicks*, ii.—What we most admire in outward features is the expression or shadow of something inward in the mind.

Addison, *Spectator*, 418.—What most recommends a description is if it represents such objects as are apt to raise a ferment in the reader's mind and to work with violence upon his passions.

Hutcheson, *Ideas of Beauty and Virtue*, IV. iv.—Everything in *Nature* can be brought to represent other things especially the passions. I. xvii.—Beauty is not in an object without relation to a perceiving mind.

Vico, *The New Science*.—Poetical statements are formed with feelings of passion and emotion.

Baumgarten, *Poetry*, 25.—Passions afford poetical ideas and it is poetical to arouse passion. 91, The predisposing causes of beautiful thinking are all passions which are not so violent as to suppress all symbolical knowledge (i.e., expression).

Home (Lord Kames), *Elements of Criticism*, II. vi.—A large object swells the heart. Sounds produce emotions or feelings that resemble them.

Reynolds, *Lectures*, xi.—Nothing, however unpromising, but may convey sentiment and produce emotion in the hands of genius.

Reid, *The Intellectual Powers*, III.—All the grandeur we ascribe to objects may be ascribed to something intellectual of which they are the signs. IV. There is hardly anything belonging to mind which may not be represented by images taken from sense, and every object of sense is beautified by borrowing from the attributes of mind.

Alison, *Nature of Taste*, Introduction.—Qualities of matter are not beautiful or sublime in themselves, but as they are the signs or expressions of qualities capable of producing emotion. I. ii. 2. It is impossible to imagine an object of taste that is not an object of emotion.

Kant, *Critique of Judgment*, 42.—Modifications of light or of sound contain a language which nature speaks to us and which seems to have an inward meaning. 59.—We call trees and buildings majestic or dignified and meadows smiling or gay; even colours are called pure, chaste, tender, because they arouse feelings.

Wordsworth, *Preface to Lyrical Ballads*.—All good poetry is the spontaneous overflow of powerful feelings. The poet has a greater power of expressing them. Poetry takes its origin from emotion recollected in tranquillity.

Coleridge, *Sound Criticism*.—The common purpose of all fine arts consists in the excitement of emotion for the immediate purpose of pleasure.

On Poesy and Art.—Art is the power of humanizing nature, of infusing the thoughts and passions of man into everything that is the object of his contemplation.

Shelley, *Defence of Poetry*.—A child at play by itself will express its delight by its voice and motions. Language is the most direct representation of the actions and passions of our internal being.

J. S. Mill, *Poetry and its Varieties*.—Poetry is the delineation of the more deep and secret workings of human emotion. Poetry is feeling, confessing itself to itself in moments of solitude and embodying itself in symbols, which are the nearest possible representations of the feeling in the exact shape in which it exists in the poet's mind.

Hegel, *Æsthetics*, Introduction iii.—In art man makes explicit to himself what he is. Art has to stir our senses, our feelings, our emotions.

Ruskin, *Modern Painters*, IV, xii, §4 (the "Pathetic Fallacy").—

> They rowed her in across the rolling foam—
> The cruel, crawling foam,

fallaciously describes foam but faithfully describes sorrow.

Hanslick, *The Beautiful in Music*, ii.—Music represents the dynamic properties of feeling.

Pater, *Style*.—Beauty is expression, the finer accommodation of speech or form or colour to a vision within, to the preferences or volitions of a soul.

R. L. Nettleship, *Lectures on Logic*.—The expression is the completed feeling, for the feeling is not fully felt till expressed, and in being expressed it is still felt but in a different way.

Bosanquet, *History of Æsthetic*.—The beautiful is what has expressiveness for sense-perception or imagination. *Three Lectures on Æsthetic*.—Feeling expressed for expression's sake. . . . A feeling so embodied in an object that it will stand still to be looked at.

Tolstoy, *What is Art?*—To evoke in oneself a feeling one has experienced, and then by movements, lines, colours, sounds or words to transmit it to others, that is art.

Santayana, *The Sense of Beauty*, 48.—The expression of passion, even of pain may constitute beauty . . . the green of spring, the bloom of youth.

Bergson, *Laughter*.—Some artists reveal to us something that cannot be translated into language, certain rhythms of life and breath that are for each individual the law of his enthusiasm and despair, his hopes and regrets.

A. C. Bradley, *Poetry for Poetry's Sake*.—When you see somebody smile, you do not apprehend separately the lines in the face which express feeling and the feeling they express. You experience the one in the other. So too when you poetically read *Hamlet*.

Croce, *Breviary of Æsthetics*, i.—Great works of art are sheer emotion absolutely identified with the most lucid imagery. ii.—Expression and beauty are not two ideas but one. *New Essays in Æsthetics*.—Every line, colour or tone is the embodiment of a mood. *Æsthetics*.—Man faced with natural beauty is the mythical Narcissus at the pool. *Problems of Æsthetics*.—What makes our hearts leap up in art and ravishes our admiration, is the passion, the fire, the feeling of the artist; if they are lacking, nothing can take their place.

Lipps, *Empathy*, *Inward Imitation*, etc.—The sensible appearance of the beautiful object is the object of æsthetic satisfaction, but its *ground* is myself. I feel myself strong, light, sure, resilient, proud *in the object*. . . . A gesture expresses to me pride or grief.

Mitchell, *Structure and Growth of the Mind*.—Shapes, curves, rhythms are naturally gay or austere, not by association but by expressiveness. The nature we find in the object depends on our past experience.

Fry, *Vision and Design*.—Rhythm of line can arouse faint echoes of emotions; when these elements are combined with the presentation of natural appearances, particularly with that of the human body, the effect is infinitely heightened.

Alexander, *Space, Time and Deity.*—We read our moods into the scene, or endow animate or inanimate objects with our feelings. We animate a statue with pride. Only through what is added to it has the beautiful object expressiveness.

Hulme, *Speculations.*—A work of art we find beautiful is an objectification of our own pleasure in activity and vitality. Geometrical art can convey intense religious emotion.

Richards, *Literary Criticism*, xviii.—What matters to the musician is not the physical connection between notes but the compatibilities and incompatibilities in the responses of emotion and attitude which they excite.

Leon, *Metaphysic of Quality.*—Art expresses, objectifies, externalizes or embodies our feelings or emotions or states of mind.

Prall, *Æsthetic Judgment*, iv–vi.—Lines, colours, sounds are expressive.

Ducasse, *Philosophy of Art*, xii. 2.—There is no sort of feeling which art may not attempt to objectify.

Gentile, *Philosophy of Art*, II. I. 7.—The artist translates into objective representations (imagery) nothing but his own feeling.

APPENDIX C
THE CORRELATION OF NATURALISTIC AND FORMAL ART SEVERALLY TO OPTIMISM AND PESSIMISM

IN T. E. Hulme's brilliant and undervalued book *Speculations*[1] the following passages occur, besides those quoted in my text.

There are two kinds of art, geometrical and vital, absolutely distinct in kind from one another. These two arts are not modifications of one and the same art but pursue different aims and are created for the satisfaction of different necessities of the mind.

Each of these arts springs from and corresponds to a certain general attitude towards the world . . . The vital art of Greece and the renaissance corresponds to a certain attitude of mind and

[1]I have quoted more fully in my *Philosophies of Beauty*.

the geometrical has always gone with a different general attitude, of greater intensity than this. . . .[1]

(Vital) art can only occur in a people whose relation to outside nature is such that it admits of a feeling of pleasure in its contemplation.[2]

Hulme speaks of primitive, Byzantine and modern art on the other hand as being geometrical, suppressing life and showing a "tendency to abstraction." He asks "What is the condition of mind of the people whose art is governed by it?" and replies "A feeling of separation in the face of outside nature. While a naturalistic art is the result of a happy pantheistic relation between man and the outside world, the tendency to abstraction, on the contrary, occurs in races whose attitude to the outside world is the exact contrary of this."[3] "In comparison with the flat and insipid optimism of the belief in progress, the new (geometrical) attitude may be in a certain sense inhuman, pessimistic."[4]

The general theory is that in ages of optimism, confidence, vitality, art will be realistic, naturalist, vital; in ages of pessimism, disillusion, fear, it will be geometrical or abstract. The first is humanist; the second mystical, religious or ascetic. Primitive men were afraid of the world; Byzantine men condemned and despised it; modern men are tired of it, and perhaps frightened too. The children of Greece and of the Renaissance were insatiably hopeful.

This is striking and captivating; it is in the grand Hegelian tradition. But, if we may mar Bacon's rhythm in the interest of modernity, "Cum multa sint in natura monodica, tamen fingit humanus intellectus dialectica."[5] When we look at actual facts we find they are not quite so simple as all that. I do not doubt that in the merest pattern which is found beautiful there is something expressive of human feeling. That,

[1]Pp. 77–8.

[2]P. 85. I have made a few emendations in the printed text, approved by the editor of Hulme's MS.

[3]Pp. 86–7.

[4]P. 93.

[5]Though much in nature is individual our mind imposes a logical pattern upon it.

I believe, is what makes it beautiful. But I am never sure how far the physical shape, the actual configuration of lines and masses and shadows and colours, determine their expressiveness for every human being or how far that depends upon the subjective elements which go to its personal interpretation. In other words, do we more resemble or differ from one another in our æsthetic appreciation of pure form? Probably, to all human eyes alike, straight lines and curves, in their purity, are severally significant of peculiar though vague experiences, but such rudimentary significance is overlaid in most men's sight by the history, meanings, associations, fashionableness, strangeness or familiarity, use, and value of what they think they are seeing, and by the mood in which they come to it. And if these "meanings" are not thought of separately, as something merely symbolized or suggested by the object, but are indistinguishably fused in its perception, they are legitimate part of the æsthetic experience.

The natural place in which we look for the facts to test the theory is England in the eighteenth and late seventeenth centuries. For there was fought out, or at least fought, a campaign in the perpetual battle between Apollo and Dionysus, or (*si libentius audiunt*) between beauty and sublimity, reason and sentiment, Greek and Gothic, classical and romantic, rule and nature, regularity and serpentine, the grand and the picturesque, the Roman and the rococo. There were skirmishes and rallies of various importance in poetry, painting, architecture, music, furnishing; but the pitched battle was in the garden. And the first thing which strikes us there is that nature, "dear," "serpentine" nature, is melancholy, sweetly, gothically melancholy, while regularity and axial design are "chearful" and "reasonably gay." Ruins are in their nature irregular, and so according to Hulme should be "vital"; but it is more noticeable to most men that they are ruins, and therefore melancholy with the sentiment of decay. Gothic is irregular, but being "monkish" it is melancholy. Classical style is regular, but since it recalls the humanistic glories of Greece, Rome and the Renaissance it is cheerful. The formal garden should have been pessimistic; but being the abode of fashion and the work of wealth, it took on a garish gaiety from which "feeling souls" fled to the irregular solace of mountains and forests, "gloomy" because haunted by poverty and danger.

Or are we then to say that such taste was an escape? That just because the period was a melancholy one, it found an antidote in the cheeriness of curvilinear nature? That, of course, turns the theory topsy-turvy, and can hardly be the truth. For these lovers of melancholy, of solitude, of the picturesque can hardly have thought the cry of their beloved owls in their beloved charnel-houses was a "merry note." They did clearly think that many if not most irregular things, including much of nature, were melancholy, and in virtue of that melancholy beautiful. Puff, in the *Critic*, "insinuates obsequious rivulets into visionary groves."

In the *Clandestine Marriage* (1766) Sterling says, "Ay, here's none of your straight lines here—but all taste—zig-zag—crinkum-crankum—in and out—right and left—so and again—twisting and turning."

Thomas Warton in the *Pleasures of Melancholy* (1747) describes, among the favourite foods of melancholy, the sky stormy or serene, the sea, forests, moss-grown piles, the owl's note, the hollow charnel. These all remind him of:

"This fleeting state of things, the vain delights."

Beattie's *Minstrel* (1771) also loved charnels and owls and winds among shuddering aisles. He was, says Dorothy Wordsworth, "much what William was when I first knew him." Coleridge thought it necessary to remind his age that:

> In nature there is nothing melancholy

for

> Ours is her wedding-garment, ours her shroud.

In 1782 Warton in a palinode retracts "the *pensive* bard's mistaken strain" which had preferred "Gothic arts" to "the just proportion and the genuine line." Beattie, writing in 1772 to Lady Forbes, says, "A mountainous country, the ocean, the sky, thoughtfulness and retirement and sometimes melancholy objects and ideas had charms in my eyes." Fletcher in 1625, Burton in 1628, Berkeley in 1713, Thomson in 1748, are all agreed that nothing is so expressive of "melancholy"—the sentiment of human littleness and transience—as ocean, mountains, forests, winding streams. Evelyn speaks of Groombridge as "a pretty melancholy seat, well wooded and watered" and unites the epithets "agreeable, melancholy and country-like" as being deserved by springs of water, cascades, rocks. Finally Pope, writing to Martha Blount about 1717, says "Nothing could have more of that melancholy which once us'd to please me (than the ride from Stonor to Oxford) . . . I rid over hanging hills, whose tops were edg'd with groves, and whose feet water'd with winding rivers, listening to the fall of Cataracts (!) below and the murmuring of winds above." Those who know the Chiltern country will be apt to think that a melancholy mood determined not only what was liked but what was seen.

To take one modern instance: Hulme was perhaps right in his presentiment that a "post-war" period would be one of disillusion. He concluded that its taste would be formal if not geometrical. But what was the picture in the Burlington House exhibition after the first world-war which transported every critic? Not the static Velasquez "Water Carrier," nor the stylized Vermeer, but the El Greco with its more than Corregiose vitality, its swirl and flutter of legs and wings and drapery and fingers.

Several alternative conclusions might emerge from such considerations:

Either the Augustans and ourselves are really a cheery crew who naturally rollick in the irregular (but against this the owls and charnels and Mr. Auden and El Greco's faces are strong): or nature and the serpentine are really gloomy things as compared with the high spirits of the parti-coloured gravel parterres at Blenheim. (But Hulme seems to prove his point that the latter is not so): or, as I am myself more disposed to conjecture, the kind of æsthetic experience which men will have in face of a given object will depend pretty little upon what it is and pretty much upon what they for the moment are, and how consequently they interpret its meaning.

Thomas Herring, Bishop of Bangor, writing in 1738 to W. Duncome of a tour in Wales, says that he was "agreeably terrified with something like the rubbish of a creation," which inclined him to "smile at the little niceties of art"; and Lord Lyttleton describing the same country in 1756 says, "The grandeur of the ocean, corresponding with that of the mountain, formed a majestic and solemn scene; ideas of immensity swelled and exalted our minds at the sight; all lesser objects appeared mean and trifling."[1]

On the other hand 1605 was probably not a period of disillusion and at any rate Bacon when he wrote *The Advancement of Learning* believed in progress. Yet he wished "the stars had been cast into some pleasant and beautiful works and orders, like the frets in the roofs of houses."

I believe that men find in patterns mainly what they put there. The glow of level sunlight may affect me with greater differences according as I think it a glorious morning or a solemn evening than according as the mountain-tops are spires or domes. Eager youth can find promise of experience alike in Chartres and in the Parthenon, as tired age can find peace and an escape in either. In 1790 Burke was probably not feeling, like Wordsworth, that "the whole world the beauty wore of promise." But even when Wordsworth's eye had learned to keep watch over man's mortality and to see our noisy years as moments in the being of the eternal silence, he did not abandon fountains, meadows, hills and groves for arabesque.

Shakespeare was a child of the Renaissance delighting, if anyone ever did, in man and the goings-on of the universe; yet, without turning his eyes from nature to geometry, he wrote of:

> Bare ruined choirs where late the sweet birds sang.

Herrick was no mystical ascetic; just because he loved life and flowers so well he could say:

[1] I owe these two quotations to Allen, *Tides in English Taste* (Harvard, 1937).

Fair daffodils, we weep to see
You haste away so soon.

. . .

We have short time to stay as you,
We have as short a spring,
As quick a growth to meet decay
As you or anything.

There is no profounder melancholy for the transience of things than in the stelai and tragedies of the Greek heyday,[1] but its melancholy is expressed not by formal or geometric style but by reference to nature; and nature is the consolation deliberately advised by Menander:

> I call him most happy who has early returned whence he came after viewing the solemn beauties of the world, the common sun, stars, water, clouds, fire. If you should live a hundred years, you will always have these before your eyes, and if but a few years, you will see nothing else more sublime than these.[2]

And it is by reference to nature that Homer had expressed the human tragedy:

> Even as the generations of leaves, such are those also of men; the wind scatters the old leaves on the earth, and the forests bud and put forth once again when the time of spring comes on. So one generation of men blooms and another fades away.[3]

And Mimnermus[4] elaborates the same simile, concluding:

> The black fates stand by, the one with the doom of dreary age, the other with the doom of death. . . . But once the appointed time of youth is past it is better to die at once than to live.

Three of the most poignant expressions of pessimism we

[1]*See* Ruskin "The Lance of Pallas" in *Modern Painters,* and Butcher "The Melancholy of the Greeks" in *Aspects of the Greek Genius.*

[2]Ὑποβολιμαῖος, Frag, 2.

[3]Iliad VI. 146.

[4]Frag, 2.

know are Greek. The first is from Theognis:[1]

It is best of all for the sons of men not to be born nor to see the bright light of the sun, and if they are born, quickly to pass the gates of Death and to lie beneath the heavy earth.

The other two are from the anthology:

I hate this unintelligible world.[2]

and

Everything that comes to pass is mockery, ashes and nothingness, for all things come from unreason.[3]

But perhaps the strongest evidence of all against Hulme is that "hope," one of the cardinal virtues of Christianity, is in Greek (ἐλπίς), when the word is unqualified, more often the name for something whose "strength lies in desperation."[4] A people which spoke thus was not confident in life.

APPENDIX D

CLASSICAL AND ROMANTIC

IN the following quotations I have italicized the words which seemed to me symptomatic.

Evelyn in his *Diary* for 1654 notes an estate which "were it approved as it might be, 'twere capable of being made a most romantiq and pleasant place."

In 1659 A. Wood in his *Life and Times* mentions "an *old* house in a romancey place . . . to refresh his mind with a *melancholy*[5] walke," and in the same year H. More in his *Immortality of the Soul* writes of "that *Imagination* which is most free, such as we use in Romantick Inventions."

[1]425.
[2]Anthol. Pal x. 96.
[3]Ibid x. 124. See Ch. XV §3.
[4]Thuc. II. lxii. 5 and cf. V. ciii.
[5]*See* Appendix C.

Boyle in 1665 speaks of "a Romantick Story," and Pepys in his *Diary* for 1666 calls Windsor "the most romantique castle that is in the world" and cites a crew who asked leave to avenge the death of their captain by a forlorn hope, "an *extraordinary* case, one of the most romantique that ever I heard of in my life and *could not have believed* . . . I could hardly abstain from *weeping*." In 1678 Cudworth in his *Intellectual System* describes the "Theology of Epicurus" as "but Romantical." In 1679 Evelyn in his *Diary* says that the Duke of Buckingham's house at Clifden is "a romantic object and altogether answers the most poetical descriptions of *solitude* . . . *imagination*." In 1685 Aubrey's *Wiltshire* says, "The *Arcadia* is about Vernditch and Wilton, and these romancey plaines and boscages did no doubt conduce to the heightening of Sir Philip Sydney's *phancie*." In 1700 a character in Rowe's *Ambitious Stepmother* apostrophizes "Dull, romantic Honour!" In 1705 Addison *On Italy* perhaps first applies the term to pure nature: "The Deserts (between Marseilles and Genoa) have been rendered famous by the penance of Mary Magdalene. . . . It is so romantic a scene . . . *irregular*, misshapen." And in 1712 in the *Spectator* No. 303 he triumphantly selects as "finely Romantick" the passage from *Paradise Lost* (I. 447):

Thammuz came next behind,
Whose annual wound in Lebanon allur'd
The Syrian damsels to lament his fate
In amorous ditties all a summer's day.
While smooth Adonis from his native rock
Ran purple to the sea suppos'd with blood
Of Thammuz yearly wounded; the love tale
Infected Sion's daughters with like heat,
Whose wanton passions in the sacred porch
Ezekiel saw, when by the vision led
His eye survey'd the dark idolatries
Of alienated Judah.

In 1716 Pope writes to Lady M. W. Montagu, "The more I examine my own mind the more romantic I find myself . . . so is everyone said to be that either admires a fine thing or praises one." In 1733 perhaps with a recollection of Addison's

Italy quoted above, he says (Moral Essays, Ep. II):

> Let then the fair one beautifully cry,
> In Magdalene's loose hair and lifted eye,
> Or dres't in smiles of sweet Cecilia shine,
> With simp'ring angels, palms and harps divine.
> . . . .
> If *folly* grow Romantic, I must paint it.

In 1726 Bishop Butler—perhaps influenced by Cudworth, quoted above—preaches in the Rolls Chapel (Sermon VI) "To make pleasure, mirth and jollity our business . . . to those who shall consider the nature of man and our condition in this life, will appear the most romantic scheme of life that ever entered in thought."

In 1736 Horace Walpole writes to Lyttleton of "a charming garden, all *wilderness*, much adapted to my Romantick inclinations," and in 1739 Gray, in a letter to his mother describes the Grande Chartreuse as "one of the most *solemn*, the most romantic, and the most *astonishing* scenes I ever beheld." In 1753 Gray writes from Durham to Mason that "All is *rude* and romantic; the sweetest spot to break your neck in or drown yourself in that ever was beheld." In the same year J. Warton in *The Adventurer* (No. 93) says that "Shakespeare has carried the romantic, the *wonderful*, the *wild*, to the most pleasing *extravagance*;" Spenser is a romantic poet.

In 1757 Sir W. Chambers on *Designs of Chinese Building* says:

> Chinese artists distinguish three different species of scenes, to which they givc the appelations of pleasing, horrid and *enchanted*. Their enchanted scenes answer in great measure to what we call *romantic*. . . . Sometimes they make a rapid torrent pass underground, the turbulent noise of which strikes the ear of the newcomer, who is at a loss to know whence it proceeds . . . impending rocks, dark *caverns*, impetuous cataracts.[1]

[1]In his *Oriental Gardening* (1772) he uses the phrase "inaccessible to the sun." In *Kubla Khan* Coleridge uses the word "sunless" as well as all those above italicized. Professor Lowes in *The Road to Xanadu* seems not to have recognized the significance of the congeniality of such a description to the poet's romantic imagination.

In 1762 Hurd in his letters on *Chivalry and Romance* asks whether there be not "something in the *Gothic* Romance peculiarly suited to the views of a *Genius*." In 1770 Gilpin in his *River Wye* calls Arthur's Seat "romantic but *not picturesque; cold, misshapen* and *uncouth*." In *Humphrey Clinker* (1771) Smollett says that at Loch Lomond, as compared with Swiss and Italian lakes, "all is *sublimity, silence* and *solitude*. Everything here is romantic." In 1771 two of the characters in Mackenzie's *Man of Feeling* come upon—

one of those figures which Salvator would have drawn. . . . The banks were covered with *fantastic* shrubwood and on one of them stood a fingerpost. . . . A rock, with some dangling wild flowers, jutted over above where the soldier lay, in which grew the stump of a large tree, white with age, and a single twisted branch shaded his face as he slept. . . . Harley found the romantic temper rising within him.[1]

In 1772 unexpected homage is offered to the rising fashion by Johnson's *Journey to the Western Isles:*

A bank such as a writer of romance might have delighted to feign. I had indeed no trees to whisper over my head but a clear rivulet streamed at my feet. The day was calm, the air soft and all was *rudeness, silence* and *solitude*. Before me and on either side were high hills which, by hindering the eye from ranging, forced the *mind to find entertainment for itself*.

In 1776 for W. Hutchinson on his *Excursion to the Lakes* "the works of Salvator Rosa express the romantic and *rocky* scene of Keswick," and Gilpin remarks in his *Highlands of Scotland* that "people call *irregular*, romantic beauties picturesque." Next year J. More calls *Thomson's Seasons* "frequently as *wild* and romantic as the pieces of Salvator." In Scott's *Autobiography* is a very significant acknowledgment, apparently referring to the year 1780, of "romantic scenery, or what afforded me at least equal pleasure, places distinguished

[1]That Harley rightly diagnosed his temper may be judged by comparison with a famous passage of the "romantic revival," Wordsworth's Prelude IV. 385 to the end of the book.

by remarkable *historical* events." In a later passage he couples *adventurous* and romantic.

We now come to what may be called the *locus classicus* for romance though it does not mention that word. The occasion was the conversion or apostasy of T. Warton caused by Reynolds' window for New College chapel in 1782:

> For long enamour'd of a barbarous age,
> A faithless truant to the *classic* page,
> Long have I lov'd to catch the simple chime
> Of minstrel-harps, and spell the fabling rhyme;
> To view the festive rites, the *knightly* play,
> That deck'd heroic Albion's *elder* day;
> To mark the mouldering halls of barons bold,
> And the *rough* castle cast in *giant* mold,
> With *gothic* manners gothic arts explore,
> And muse on the magnificence of *yore.*
>
> . . . .
>
> Sudden the *sombrous* imagery is fled,
> Which late my *visionary rapture* fed;
> Thy powerful hand has broke the gothic chain
> And brought my bosom back to *truth* again,
>
> . . . .
>
> To *truth*, whose charms deception's *magic* quell,
> And bind coy *fancy* in a stronger spell.

SUGGESTED BOOKS AND PASSAGES

MOST of the works mentioned are quoted, and where necessary translated, in my *Philosophies of Beauty from Socrates to Robert Bridges*.

§ indicates introductory works.

* indicates works of philosophical or historic importance.

The lists are approximately chronological.

A
THE HISTORICAL AUTHORITIES

Plato §	*Hippias Major*.
*	*Republic*, 400–2, 597–607.
*§ Aristotle	*Poetics*, IV, VI, VII, IX.
*Longinus	*On the Sublime*, XXXV, XXXIX.
Addison	*Spectator*, 411–14, 418, 420, 421.
*Hume	*Treatise of Human Nature*, II. i. 8, ii. 5.
	Essay XXIII, *The Standard of Taste*.
*Burke	*The Sublime and Beautiful*.
*Kant	*Critique of Judgment*, §§1–11, 14–17, 23, 25, 28.
*§ Wordsworth	*Preface to Lyrical Ballads* (1800).
	Essay Supplementary to Preface (1815).
*Schopenhauer	*The World as Will and Idea*, III, §§38–52.
	Supplement, Chapter XXIX.
*Hegel	*Æsthetics* (Introduction).
§ Tolstoy	*What is Art?*

B
CONTEMPORARY BOOKS

Santayana	*The Sense of Beauty*.
*Bergson	*Laughter*.
*§ A. C. Bradley	*Poetry for Poetry's Sake* (in "Oxford Lectures").
*Croce	*Essentials of Æsthetic* (*Breviario*).

* Lipps	*Einfühlung, innere Nachahmung und Organempfindungen* (in "Archiv für die Gesamte Psychologie, i, iv).
Clive Bell	*Art*
R. Fry	*Vision and Design.*
Alexander	*Beauty and Other Forms of Value.*
Hulme	*Speculations.*
Richards	*Principles of Literary Criticism.*
§ Carritt	*What is Beauty?*
* Collingwood	*Principles of Art.*

C
BOOKS OF REFERENCE

Bosanquet	*History of Æsthetics*
Carritt	*Theory of Beauty.*
Croce	*Æsthetics*, Part II (2nd edition of translation by D. Ainslie).
Robertson	*Genesis of Romantic Theory.*
§ Hussey	*The Picturesque.*

INDEX

For Product Safety Concerns and Information please contact our EU representative GPSR@taylorandfrancis.com Taylor & Francis Verlag GmbH, Kaufingerstraße 24, 80331 München, Germany

Batch number: 10725863

Printed by Printforce, the Netherlands